TRUSTING PERFORMANCE

Cognitive Studies in Literature and Performance

Trusting Performance

A Cognitive Approach to Embodiment in Drama

Naomi Rokotnitz

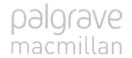

First published in 2011 by
PALGRAVE MACMILLAN®
in the United States—a division of St. Martin's Press LLC,
175 Fifth Avenue, New York, NY 10010.

Where this book is distributed in the UK, Europe and the rest of the world,
this is by Palgrave Macmillan, a division of Macmillan Publishers Limited,
registered in England, company number 785998, of Houndmills,
Basingstoke, Hampshire RG21 6XS.

Palgrave Macmillan is the global academic imprint of the above companies
and has companies and representatives throughout the world.

Palgrave® and Macmillan® are registered trademarks in the United States,
the United Kingdom, Europe and other countries.

ISBN: 978–0–230–33737–4

Library of Congress Cataloging-in-Publication Data

Rokotnitz, Naomi.
    Trusting performance : a cognitive approach to embodiment in drama /
Naomi Rokotnitz.
        p. cm.—(Cognitive studies in literature and performance)
    Includes bibliographical references.
    ISBN 978–0–230–33737–4 (hardback)
    1. Drama—History and criticism. 2. Drama—Psychological aspects.
3. Human body in literature. 4. Characters and characteristics in literature.
5. Performance—Psychological aspects. I. Title.

PN1631.R55 2011
792—dc23   2011017480

A catalogue record of the book is available from the British Library.

Design by Newgen Imaging Systems (P) Ltd., Chennai, India.

First edition: December 2011

10 9 8 7 6 5 4 3 2 1

Printed and bound in Great Britain by
CPI Antony Rowe, Chippenham and Eastbourne

To Herbert, Jacqueline, Jonathan, Daniel, and Lia with unconditional love.

Contents

Acknowledgments

This book is an updated and greatly extended continuation of the PhD dissertation I began at Bar Ilan University in 2001. I wish to thank the university for awarding me the Presidential Scholarship for Outstanding Doctoral Students and for employing me thereafter. I wish to express my gratitude and affection for Professor Ellen Spolsky, advisor, mentor, friend, and inspiration, founding godmother of the discipline now termed "cognitive approaches to literature," for her challenging, rigorous, and ever-ready attentiveness. I thank my many marvellous teachers: Jean Gooder, Sue Manning, Germaine Greer, Stephan Collini, Caroline Walmsley, Graham Banks, Tim Williams, Ruth Whiting, Graham Noble, Colin Prowse, Dennis Archer, Alan Gent, Kinereth Mayer; and my fierce and discerning editors Vera Glasberg, Jerome Mandel and John Lutterbie. Special thanks to Bruce McConachie, who expressed faith in this project in its infancy and secured a home for its publication. To Iris Dahan, who taught me how to listen for embodied signals. To Samantha Hasey and Joel Breuklander from Palgrave Macmillan. To Rohini Krishnan from Newgen Publishing and Data Services. To Elizabeth Hart, Lisa Zunshine, Alan Richardson, Amy Cook and Rhonda Blair, among other literary scholars committed to this interdisciplinary venture, who have paved the academic road for this book.

To my wise and wonderful mother, Jacqueline Rokotnitz; to my talented brother, Jonathan Rokotnitz, who also contributed the evocative cover illustration; to my sparkle-eyed children, Daniel and Lia; and in memory of my beloved father, Herbert.

To John Keats for his invitation to "burst joy's grape against [our] palate[s] fine."

Introduction

Ha, ha, what a fool Honesty is! And
Trust, his sworn brother, a very simple gentleman
(The Winter's Tale IV.iv 600)

"Man conquers himself not in any detached freedom of standing over
against the world, but rather in his daily intercourse with the world, in
allowing himself to participate in its conditionedness. Only by doing so
does he attain the proper attitude for the act of knowing"
(Gadamar 1947: 16)

Most people have experienced a significant betrayal at least once in their lives. We extended our friendship, love and trust and received in return a slap in the face or, worse, a stab in the back. People can often be selfish, manipulative, dishonest and deliberately hurtful. And yet people also regularly place their trust in others and cooperate with "genetically unrelated strangers [and] with individuals they will never meet again" (Krueger et al. 2007: 3).[1] Are we all "very simple" fools? Or willfully blind? Or is there an advantage to trusting that exceeds the potential risk of error?

I. Orientation

In the quest for reliable knowledge, we must repeatedly confront the frustrating realization that there are a great many things we cannot know for certain. Human comprehension is contingent and provisional. It would indeed be foolish to object to a measure of humility in our interactions with, and interpretations of, the world around us and the people with whom we come into contact. Logical analysis convinces us, more often than not, that the best defense against error and disappointment is the cultivation of both skepticism regarding knowledge and vigilant suspicion of others. However, the inclination to trust and the feelings of well-being and security it generates are not governed by logic. Thankfully, trust is an embodied aptitude.

Embodied modes of reception and perception are those that do not require logical analysis for their verification; their presence and effects are made manifest in the body. These include sense-perception, emotional responsiveness, memory, intuition, and imagination. The capacity to pay closer attention to the evidence provided by *embodied knowledge* is foundational to an understanding of the multiple ways with which we interact with our environment. As Shaun Gallagher and Dan Zahavi assert,

> Bodily behavior, expression, and action are essential to (and not merely contingent vehicles of) some basic forms of consciousness. Mental states do not simply serve to explain behaviour; rather, some mental states are directly apprehended in the bodily expressions of people whose mental states they are. (2008: 148)

Some experiences are registered in our actively analyzing conscious minds; others write themselves into the very fibers of our physical selves.[2]

In this book I will argue that it is precisely this experiential, embodied knowledge that provides the basis for the fostering of trust. Though reasons for doubt are ever present, there *are* truths of which we may be sufficiently satisfied in order to trust with confidence, and these truths are usually those that are apprehended and confirmed in the body.

Acknowledging that individual identities are influenced by specificities of historical context, gender, ethnicity, education, economic status, and physical (dis)abilities, the definition of "body" in this book encompasses the physical traits that appear to be universally human. This is not a prescriptive definition of normativity, but an acknowledgment that most humans stand on two legs and experience the world as vertical beings. As Lakoff and Johnson explore at length in *Metaphors We Live By*, the linguistic constructions that denote up-down, front-back orientation derive from the physical experience of the embodied creatures we are.

As the title *Trusting Performance* indicates, the central aim of this book is twofold. First, to celebrate the human propensity to trust—in ourselves, in others, and in our ability to make diverse subject positions intelligible to one another. This advantageous propensity is, I maintain, facilitated by physical communication. I therefore examine embodied resonance and its role in personal experience and interpersonal communication. Second, I explore how drama both enacts and teaches the value of learning through and from our bodies. Drama presents the tangible actions of living bodies on stage to living bodies in the audience. In addition to—and by no means instead of—the intellectual stimulation of the narrative argument and its linguistic dimensions, dramatic performance arouses and co-opts both performers' and audiences' embodied receptiveness, thereby facilitating a deep emotional learning that can bypass resistance, bias, and fear, often opening new avenues for communication and encouraging trust. [3] Attending a theater performance is anything but a passive undertaking.

I use the term "drama" to denote both the texts of the plays studied in this book and the processes of their production and performance. The plays have been deliberately chosen for their diversity, each chapter considering a different play, dramatic genre, historical period, philosophical context, and creative approach. And yet, I locate in each a crucial and defining reverence for embodied knowledge. This task calls for an interdisciplinary approach to epistemological inquiry: a cognitive approach to drama.

Cognition, at its simplest, defines "the processing of information entering the brain from the outside world through sensory portals" (Cromwell and Panksepp 2011: 43).[4] However, because the term is often used as "a moniker for practically all the interesting functions the brain performs to facilitate behavioral adaptations and survival" (46–48), it has been subjected to some overuse and even misuse, particularly with regard to theories of "the biopsychology of attention, emotions and motivations" (49–51).[5] My use of the term cognition, discussed at length below, follows the work of philosophers Mark Johnson and Andy Clark and entails a situated, embodied, dynamic system of networks, including pre-conscious body-brain functions and affective states, as well as conscious discursive analysis and environmental aids. Distinct functions receive due attention in the pages that follow, but the emphasis returns again and again to evidence of the highly interactive nature of all human cognitive mechanisms. I contend that by acknowledging our physical architecture and the paradigms instantiated by our biological makeup, we not only discover a natural propensity to connectivity, but also begin to reconfigure our notions of knowledge in terms of collaborative effort. Since the dynamic of reciprocal interaction in dramatic performance both mimics and complicates this propensity, drama provides a fecund testing ground for exploring this process.

II. Embodiment, Relationality, and Connectivity

Despite the tradition that, since Plato, located the site of knowledge in our conscious, reasoning faculties, contemporary philosophers, biologists, psychologists and neurologists are converging on the recognition that bodily knowledge is foundational to understanding. There have always been those who insisted upon the value of bodily knowledge.[6] But it is only since the phenomenological turn in philosophy at the beginning of the twentieth century, and in light of recent advances in science in the last three decades, that Andy Clark, for example, can assert that our cognitive profile is "essentially the profile of an embodied and situated organism" (Clark 1998: 273); the brain is "just a part (albeit a crucial and special part) of a spatially and temporally extended process" of cooperation between brain, body, and environmental aids (271). Mark Johnson concurs by arguing that, as mind and body are "not separate and distinct ontological kinds," the "classical representational theory of mind," must be replaced by "an account of embodied meaning that emerges as structures of organism-environment interactions or transactions" (Johnson 2007: xii).

The long-standing belief in the division between body and mind was traditionally accompanied by a prioritizing of reason over emotion. This bias must also be corrected. Neurologist Antonio Damasio concedes that emotions precede reason, but asserts that this chronology does not determine the relative value of each capacity. Our initial response to stimuli is physical and rarely voluntary, while the secondary process of conscious deliberation and reflection upon these responses follows later (Damasio 1999: 283). This suggests that we may experience emotions without reason but that reason is exercised only after emotion is experienced, rendering reason and emotion equally integral to decision making (41). Intelligent behavior requires critical reasoning that fully acknowledges our multifarious emotional compass.

Consider, for example, pleasant and unpleasant smells, causing the emotions of pleasure or disgust respectively. Though seeming to be opposite responses, both pleasant and unpleasant smells are processed by the orbitofrontal cortex, the brain region responsible for the olfactory sense. However the intensity of our response, ranging from mildly to violently affected, is processed by a different brain region (the amygdala). This suggests that the registration of emotion in the brain is comprised of two factors: intensity (arousal levels) and valence (degree of pleasure). But the impact of each factor is often determined by pre-conditioned biological preferences. For instance, unpleasant stimuli tend to be more arousing and affect us more powerfully than pleasant stimuli, "likely reflecting the greater adaptive importance of avoiding potential harm" (Hamann 2003:107). This arousal may be registered in BOLD (blood-oxygen-level-dependency) signals without particular neurons firing (Phillips et al. 2004: 1491; Moll et al. 2005: 68).

This relatively recent discovery ought to have a formidable effect upon all epistemological inquiry, for it demonstrates the ease with which our (pre)dispositions, emotional responses, and memory may be affected on a pre-conscious level. Even more important, we may never become conscious of this affective conditioning; we may proceed with our lives, having made a crucial decision, without ever knowing what prompted us to make that decision. Advertisers and propagandists have been manipulating subliminal messages for decades but it is time to acknowledge that, in our daily interactions, what counts as knowledge should be radically revised. As Katherine Hayles writes, "conscious thought becomes as it were the epiphenomenon corresponding to the phenomenal base the body provides" (Hayles 1993: 161).

Furthermore, though rational thought takes place in the frontal cortex, rationality is not exclusively in possession of that cortex. Psychologist Jonathan Haidt suggests, "the orbitofrontal cortex appears to be a better candidate for the id, or for St. Paul's flesh, than for the superego or the spirit" (Haidt 2006: 11). Haidt's "Promethean account" of the evolution of the human brain[7] suggests that the sensation of having a separate, ethereal self, which is somehow detached from one's body, is itself generated by the biochemistry of that same body. Complex thought patterns, reason, faith, and the apprehension of what we term "the spiritual," are inextricably bound to our flesh and to our pre-conscious, pre-verbal, physical drives.

Nonetheless, the suggestion that all cognition is embodied does not imply that all abstract conceptions are generated by motor mechanisms; the embodied cognition hypothesis is not so reductive. As Clark remarks, it seems likely that humans learn through interaction with their environment, having evolved to exploit "any mixture of neural, bodily, and environmental resources, along with their complex, looping, often nonlinear interactions" (1998: 259) in order to inform and supplement understanding, as well as compensate for limitations. Interaction appears to be the defining characteristic of embodied cognition.[8]

For instance, neuropsychological research over the last three decades points to the conclusion that human perception of actions is also influenced by the implicit knowledge of the central nervous system concerning the movements that it itself is capable of producing. To a great extent, we are able to interpret the actions of others because we share their motor schemata—we share a bodily knowledge of them. The neurologist Vittorio Gallese terms this "motor equivalence" (Gallese 2001: 47). Gallese argues that humans are endowed with a mirror-matching capacity, an inborn inclination to imitate, indeed simulate, actions they observe others perform. Mirror-matching appears to be "a basic organizational feature of the brain" (46). Mimicry is defined as the tendency to synchronize affective expressions, vocalizations, postures, and movements with those of another person (Singer & Lamm, 2009). Simulation describes the internal replication of observed action through bodily mechanisms that do not require conscious thought or reflection, but rely upon a shared "brain-body system" (Gallese, Keysers, and Rizzolati 2004: 397).

Motor theories of cognition have a long history in psychology, dating back at least to Berkeley's (1709) motor interpretation of depth perception, and have been proposed as explanations for a wide range of mental processes.[9] The current explosion of interest in such theories is related to, though not wholly dependant upon, the discovery in the early 1990s of mirror neurons, deemed by many "one of the most important findings in neuroscience" in recent years (Zak 2007: 1158).[10] According to this hypothesis, primates and humans possess a set of neurons that are activated by goal-related behaviors. They do not respond to random movements, such as the movement of waves upon the sea surface, but only to the apprehension of meaningful interaction, such as a hand suddenly reaching out from those waves. When we observe an action we perceive to be intentional, or meaningful, our mirror neurons activate both the visual areas that observe the action and, concurrently, recruit the motor circuits used to perform that action—the circuits that we would use were we to perform that action ourselves. Giacomo Rizolatti and Michael Arbib (1998) explain further that this mirror matching is involuntary. Even though we are able to resist imitating actions we observe others perform, we are not able to prevent our bodies from responding at the preconscious level of simulation. As Gallese notes, "action observation implies action simulation" (2001: 37).

Mirror neurons appear to participate in human action-recognition and to influence motor memory. But the leading neurologists in this field agree that mirror neurons cannot function by themselves. Instead, these neurons work in conjunction with other neural networks, such as those responsible for memory and inference, and also with an intricate network of peripheral nervous system pathways stretching all over the body, activating "motor equivalence." [11] The Mirror Neuron System (MNS) is part of a larger system of "convergence-divergence zones" (CDZs), which are neural ensembles that collect information separately but rely upon mutually dependant feedback loops. Thus, any response to them results from a coalition of forces.[12]

Although there are a great many things we do not know about our brains, it appears the human cognitive system is best described as a holistic coalition of interacting cerebral and bodily mechanisms. As cognitive neuropsychologists Bradford Z. Mahon and Alfonso Caramazza state:

> The activation of the sensory and motor systems during conceptual processing serves to ground 'abstract' and 'symbolic' representations in the rich sensory and motor content that mediates our physical inter-action with the world. (Mahon and Caramazza 2008: 68)

Thus, sensory and motor information contributes to and supplements the creation of representational concepts and complements the generality and flexibility of abstract and symbolic conceptual representations. Similarly, social cognition, assert Keysers and Gazzola, relies equally upon simulation and reflection, intuition and analysis.[13]

The processes by which we expand our knowledge rely upon multiple sources of information, through which we apprehend varied and often contradictory inputs, and to which we then respond, both consciously and unconsciously, through intricate physical and psychological mechanisms. These responses are then open to interpretation and re-interpretation, and are susceptible to adjustment, adaptation, supplementation, and change, extending that which Clark terms our "cognitive scaffolding" (1998: 274).

This scaffolding is constructed, reinforced, and integrated in different ways by different people and their individual bodies. As Charlotte Ross has noted,

> Our condition as embodied subjects is profoundly inflected by the relationship between mind and body, psyche and soma, consciousness and fleshy matter, which may be perceived or experienced in multitudinous ways, from profound integration to definitive separation of these elements. [. . .] each different manifestation of the borders of the physical body [. . .] is charged with significance. (Ross 2011: 2, 14)

Moreover, it must be noted that on an hourly basis, biotechnological advances make bodily modifications and substitutions more prevalent, continually extending our conception of embodiment.[14]

However, I am primarily concerned with the cognitive potentialities of organic human bodies and the faculties they share with other human bodies, particularly those that give rise to personhood and enable empathy.[15] Social neuroscientists have found that sharing the emotions of others is associated with the automatic, involuntary activation of the same neural structures that are active during the first-hand experience of that emotion, further enriching the mirror-resonance hypothesis. This synchronized resonance often also enables us to "understand what it feels like when someone else experiences sadness or happiness, and also pain, touch, or tickling" (Singer et al. 2004: 1157), creating emotional correlation or contagion, (the communication of one's mood to others) (Keen 2006: 209).[16] However, recent studies also show that empathy is a highly flexible phenomenon and that "vicarious responses are malleable with respect to a number of factors—such as contextual appraisal, the interpersonal relationship between empathizer and other, or the perspective adopted during observation of the other" (Singer and Lamm 2009: 81).

Thus, empathy necessarily involves body-based simulation that provides "experiential insights into other minds" (Gallese, Keysers, and Rizzolati 2004: 401); but empathy is not sufficient in itself to decode these minds. In order to attempt such decoding, we require conscious analysis. Some refer to this secondary, discursive skill as Theory of Mind (ToM). According to this theory, humans assume that others have a mental and emotional life more or less comparable to their own and thereby infer other individuals' intentionality. The proponents of ToM hold that it is this skill that allows us to identify and contemplate mental states in others, and to interpret these states in terms of beliefs, goals, intentions, and emotions (Agnew 2007).[17] However, the term ToM is somewhat misleading. The word theory conjures structured, conscious processing, the consideration of logical inferences and the relations between them. Yet, in the introduction to *Theory of Mind and Literature* (2011), Paula Leverage, Howard Mancing, and their colleagues claim that ToM includes mind reading, empathy, and the "creative imagination of another's perspective" (Leverage et al. 2011). This suggests that their use of the term "empathy" is broader than the scientific definition I adopt in this book and includes the kind of sympathetic emotional contagion which Jonathan Levy and Jean Decety separate from empathy (discussed at length in Chapter 4).

Whatever the mechanisms involved, the process of thinking and theorizing about the mental states of others is particularly relevant when we seek to establish grounds for mutual goodwill. In such cases, we must infer each other's intentions to determine whether or not to trust and whether or not our partner(s) will reciprocate this trust in the future (Kreuger et al. 2007: 6). Nonetheless, it must be stated upfront that empathy and/or effective ToM do not by any means guarantee sympathy. Decety defines empathy as "the ability to appreciate the emotions and feelings of others with a minimal distinction between self and other" and sympathy as "feelings of concern about the welfare of others" (Decety 2010: 1). As the history of torture attests, empathy can exist without sympathy. However, although the involuntary, physical, mirror-resonance that defines empathy need not necessarily lead to sympathy, sympathy is best achieved through eliciting empathy.[18] And that is a topic I address in depth in Chapters 3 and 4.

III. Impact on Literary Studies

If relationality and connectivity are imprinted into our very cognitive makeup—a modular system, made up of highly specialized and yet intricately interconnected networks of extended reciprocity—why should scholars not adopt the same model and foster interdisciplinary collaboration?[19] An increasing number of scholars are finding it productive to enrich their own field of expertise with theoretical, methodological, and empirical data gleaned from other fields. Synthesis, coherence, and cross-fertilization do not promise watertight answers; neither do they imply amateur reductionism.

Cognitive literary studies arose in response to the conviction that we may gain a great deal by "the blending of humanistic and scientific discourses as long as we are careful about how we bring the approaches together and about what we can expect their blending to reveal" (Jackson 2003: 191). Ever since Johnson and Lakoff's *Metaphors We Live By* (1980) and Johnson's *The Body in The Mind* (1987) challenged previous interpretations of language construction and the human conditions they represent, literary critics have been inspired to apply the findings of cognitive scientists to the interpretation of literary texts.[20] Pioneers in the field, such as Mark Turner, Ellen Spolsky, F. Elizabeth Hart, Patrick Colm Hogan, Alan Richardson, and Lisa Zunshine, do not expect science to validate or provide indisputable evidence for their literary claims but, rather, to point towards key issues, particularly regarding cognition, that may be equally illuminated by a number of disciplines.[21]

Scientific findings allow literary critics to extend the scope of their analyses while, at the same time, complementing and supplementing scientific investigations, enriching the feedback loops of epistemological inquiry. This book presents recent discoveries in psychology, neurology, cognitive linguistics, and philosophy of mind that support intuitive claims for the transformative possibilities of dramatic performance, drawing together literary scholars, theater practitioners, philosophers, psychologists, and cognitive scientists.

IV. Dramatic Performance and Accessing Embodied Receptiveness

The scientific findings and critical approach briefly outlined above are particularly pertinent to theater studies. The same embodied mechanisms that ground intersubjective communication and mind reading are also responsible for our readiness to engage with fictional agents. Lisa Zunshine has demonstrated how "our ability to navigate multiple levels of intentionality" in a narrative both extends and challenges our capacity to identify with and to analyze others, making literary texts a source of valuable training and knowledge (2003: 8). Following John Dewey, Mark Johnson has argued that aesthetic contemplation of the arts provides "heightened, intensified and highly integrated experiences of meaning, using all our ordinary resources of meaning-making" and, thus, "we can find no better examples of how meaning happens than by attending to the arts" (2007: xii–xiii).

I suggest that drama, through facilitating the interaction of audiences with actor-characters in performance, offers the most productive environment in which to test these hypotheses. Indeed, in their preface to *Mirrors in the Brain: How Our Minds Share Action and Emotion*, neurophysiologist Giacomo Rizzolatti and philosopher Corrado Sinigaglia cite director Peter Brook, who commented that neuroscience has finally

> started to understand what has long been common knowledge in the theater: the actor's efforts would be in vain if he were not able to surmount all cultural and linguistic barriers and share his bodily sounds and movements with the spectators, who thus actively contribute to the event and become one with the players on stage. (Rizzolatti and Sinigaglia 2006: ix)

The word "theater" is cognate with "theory;" the Greek *theatron*, is a derivation of *thea*, "a sight" and of *theasthai*, "to view," which are related to *theorema*, "spectacle" and "speculation." Theater audiences speak of going to see a play and conceive of the experience, first and foremost, as viewers. Vision has indeed long been recognized as the pre-eminent sense with which we perceive but, as explained above, scientists have recently shown that vision permeates the body: seeing is a form of active engagement with external stimuli that resonates within.[22] In addition to the levels of symbolic understanding that invite audiences to infer multiple levels of meanings in the play, audiences also benefit from their embodied engagement with audio-visual effects and, most importantly, the bodies of actors in performance. As Bruce McConachie acknowledges in *Engaging Audiences*, from the point of view of cognitive studies, there are "fundamental differences between readers making sense of signs on a printed page and the mostly nonsymbolic activity of spectator cognition" (McConachie 2008: 3). Spectatorship is a form of action and interaction, "more proactive than the traditions of semiotics, behaviorism, and Freudianism have generally understood" (4).

Drama differs further from other literary genres in that its performance necessarily limits the hermeneutic possibilities of its text(s). Directorial choices determine the way in which the text is uttered and interpreted by those on stage, while acoustic and visual codes further influence semiotic analysis. Drama is therefore always two-directional, juggling stability (the text) with variability (individual productions).[23] But each production creates a microcosm in which actors and audience members participate in a reciprocal experience. This is not to say that a uniform response to production or performance could ever be achieved, or that it is even desirable, but that such experiences access the body directly, teaching it that, despite multiple discursive arguments to the contrary, shared understanding is not only possible but also common. Moreover, the production and performance of plays in itself necessitates collaborative teamwork, which in turn reinforces a confidence in communication among the writer(s), director(s), producer(s), performer(s) and audience(s), encouraging the embodied understanding that leads to trust.

V. The Moral Dimension: Freedom of Choice

The paradigm of connectivity allows us to begin to reconfigure notions of knowledge and identity, and also of community and moral accountability. Though biology and culture largely determine the range of possibilities available to the individual subject, I believe that each subject nonetheless has a range of options from which to choose, and which constitute that subject's personal, moral, aesthetic, and political responsibility.

Beginning with the infant engaging the mother's glance, our store of knowledge alters as we alter, is changed, adapted, disregarded, or reinforced in relation to our ever-expanding experiential engagement with the world. But that world does not predetermine all our choices and (inter)actions. Knowledge is not gained through a process of open reception to any and all input but, rather, arises from a self-organized set of object-and/or *goal-oriented activities* (Clark 1998: 276). This means that sensation is processed by the brain in relation to its action potential; we select the relevant input that directs our behavior in the world. We must, therefore, take responsibility for those choices.

Knowledge and meaning are neither open to infinite proliferation nor are they fully determined. Within the (restricted) biological, cultural and social environments in which we exist, we can avail ourselves of the possibility for individual action and exercise both moral responsibility and personal creativity. As Stoppard argues in *Travesties* (Chapter 2 of this book), not all individuals have the same creative talent. But, as Wertenbaker argues in *Our Country's Good* (Chapter 3), at each stage in our lives, there are windows of opportunity that afford us the possibility of choice. I aim to show that, while change may often arise from involuntary, pre-conscious response mechanisms that affect somatic identity irrespective of conscious choice, nonetheless, if we are attuned to our bodies and recognize changes as they occur, we may accommodate them, adapt accordingly, own and direct their potential influence or, alternately, reject them.[24]

VI. Arrangement

This project began as a search for evidence to support my intuitive attraction to and sympathy with those who have the courage to trust. Of the abundance of materials I encountered, those I found by far the most compelling and persuasive were plays. Rational contemplation inevitably leads to doubt; philosophy generates suspicion. But while doubt is necessary for rigorous analysis, and essential for the advancement of intelligent inquiry, art and drama can also teach us of other forms of knowing that are no less valid, rigorous, or true. Doubt is important for our survival; trust is important for our mental and emotional wellbeing.

Not all plays lead to trust; some deliberately aim to undermine it. But each play studied in this book presents its own challenge to radical skepticism and relativism, and presents its own justification of trust.[25] As explained above, the modes of expression deployed by dramatists— the means by which they may access both actors and audiences' conscious and pre-conscious mechanisms of cognition and create a charged experiential event—render the impact of dramatic production particularly powerful. The four plays discussed in each of the following chapters have been chosen for their distinct approaches to skepticism and their unique responses to it through celebrating existence and encouraging trust in embodied receptiveness. Each play also, significantly, presents a different set of arguments for the role of drama in such an endeavor.

My chief interest in this book lies in contemporary culture and the English language. With these parameters in mind, I begin with an Early Modern play that defines many of the concerns that continued into the Modern era, and proceed chronologically to the present day. The focus-text of Chapter 1 is Shakespeare's *The Winter's Tale* (1610), which responds to the climate of doubt generated by the Renaissance, Reformation, and Counter-Reformations. Stoppard's *Travesties* (1974), in Chapter 2, sets out to make a self-reflexive comment about Postmodern culture in relation to, and as a revision of, high Modernism. In Chapter 3, Wertenbaker's *Our Country's Good* (1988), produced during the Thatcher-Regan era, harks back to eighteenth century Enlightenment and Sentimentalist models of civic life. In Chapter 4, *33 Variations* (2008), drawing upon Romantic and Existentialist theories, emphasizes the centrality of personal choice in attitudes to both doubt and trust.

The effectiveness of different dramatic genres and of attitudes to performance is also examined. Chapter 1 studies a tragicomedy, which seeks to defy skepticism through legitimizing multiple forms of knowledge acquisition, suggesting that trust is established through informed and conscious choice. Chapter 2 examines a parody, which connects linguistic and intertextual theories of relationality with embodied affects and performance strategies. Chapter 3 analyzes a postmodern comedy that presents theatrical experience itself as a means of articulating both personal and social identity, (re)creating community, love, and trust. Chapter 4 is not modeled on conventional dramatic categories but upon the variation form in music; its cumulative, evolving harmonies, merge history with fantasy, music with drama, and physical pain with spiritual elevation to celebrate flexibility, innovation, and inspiration.

In addition to their thematic connections, the chapters are further connected by an overarching cognitive argument that is clarified and strengthened as the book progresses. As outlined above, cognition studies suggest that humans have evolved to make connections between disparate objects and people, creating for ourselves multiple communities (biological, cultural, linguistic, ideological), complementing and extending the insights offered by dramatic productions. As the evolutionary geneticist and zoologist Richard Lewontin insists, "Organisms do not find the world in which they develop. They make it. Reciprocally, the internal forces are not autonomous, but act in response to the external" (Lewontin 1991: 63). In place of the sectarian divisions, suspicion, and cynicism that characterized much of late twentieth century philosophy and culture—considered in Chapter 2—we may now avail ourselves of a broad spectrum of varied fields of knowledge, which together suggests hat, far from being isolated individuals trapped in private cells/hells, we have adapted to make use of shared, interactive processes. Drama is a particularly rewarding example of such processes.

Chapter 1

"It Is Required You Do Awake Your Faith": Learning to Trust the Body through Performing *The Winter's Tale*

First performed during the turbulent Reformation crisis of faith, Shakespeare's *The Winter's Tale* encourages doubt in the form of intelligent questioning that counterweighs both blind faith and tyranny—a form of prudent skepticism. At the same time, the play fights off the destructive lure of unqualified skepticism, which in its extremity encourages radical relativism and nihilism. *The Winter's Tale* demonstrates that unqualified skepticism leads to self-betrayal: the destruction of both family and kingdom. But it is a matter of wisdom and measure to understand that skepticism of the prudent kind is not only reasonable but also productive.

Shakespeare's advocacy of both mystery and boundary fluidity is expressed in the strange generic fusion of the play: a tragicomic pastoral romance. Stanley Cavell's description of tragedy as presenting "a response to skepticism" (Cavell 1987: 5) provides a framework for studying the tragic first half of the play, in which King Leontes exaggerates the imagined betrayal of his trust to a level that involves conceptual extinction of the whole world. In the second half of the play, a romance-structure leads to comic resolution. Leontes's (philosophical) doubt is defeated by Perdita-Natural-Knowing and Hermione-Grace/faith. The tragic consequences of the denial of embodied receptiveness are overcome (almost) when Leontes learns that human control against error lies in awareness rather than logic and stubborn dogmatism. This conclusion is reached through deploying a pastoral structure, in defiance of Reformation suspicion of sense perception.

By engaging with Leontes's learning process, Shakespeare's audience is encouraged to value flexibility: balancing doubt with trust, logic with sense-perception, judgment with compassion. Finally, Hermione's famous resurrection scene—in which a statue comes to life—is explained through acknowledging Shakespeare's confidence in his audience's attunement to embodied receptiveness.

Chapter 2

"Reason in Madness": a Doubling of Immortality in Tom Stoppard's *Travesties*

In this chapter I suggest that Stoppard builds upon the innately intertextual nature of both language and art through a wonderfully funny parody of a specifically postmodern brand, thereby providing a model for an interconnected world that may defy radical relativism. *Travesties* (1974) complements the understanding that humans are biologically predisposed to perceive the world in terms of relationality and connectivity. It also demonstrates that part of the journey towards defying the skeptical paralysis that characterizes much of postmodern thought involves a containment of what Owen Miller terms the potential "promiscuity" of the proliferation of meaning (Miller 1985: 25). Stoppard's intertextual-parody opens up productive communication channels between texts, intertexts, history and art, artists and audiences; polysemy is encouraged but total abandonment is not. Stoppard convinces us that humans are not doomed to lonely isolation and solipsism. Rather, as scientists argue more adamantly every day, we are responsive individuals who operate within multiple interpretive communities, through which we make sense of things, predict, communicate, and create. Ultimately, *Travesties* promises its characters and creator a "doubling of immortality" (*Travesties* 42) of the kind promised the lovers in Shakespeare's "Sonnet 18."

Chapter 3

Staging Change and Conciliation in Timberlake Wertenbaker's *Our Country's Good*

Our Country's Good dramatizes the events that led to a performance of George Farquhar's *The Recruiting Officer* by a group of transported convicts in Australia in 1789. Wertenbaker displays the heated discussions, confrontations, and violent interruptions that precede this public performance, as well as the remarkable effects of cooperation, empathy, and self-articulation that emerge during rehearsals.

Wertenbaker argues thereby for the power of dramatic performance to reconstruct damaged spirits and transform a heterogeneous, hostile group of individuals into a civil community in which respect, trust, and affection are possible.

The play's preoccupation with language and texts complements the themes of Stoppard's *Travesties* (Chapter 2). The seemingly miraculous effects of the production of Farquhar's play, set against the realities of human subjugation and debasement, relate to Shakespeare's treatment of the magic of theatrical experience in *The Winter's Tale* (Chapter 1). Crucially, the play within the play re-creates trust through correcting embodied experience: the participants' bodies are in effect re-programmed. The play's ultimate success, as in *The Winter's Tale* and *Travesties,* depends on a celebration and affirmation of the power of words and of performance to defy radical skepticism and despair, and to (re)create trust.

Wertenbaker thereby also dramatizes many of the premises of the Enlightenment, among them contractual political theories and Sentimentalist moral theories, the combination of which suggests a powerful counterforce to despair. These premises are extended by drama, as Wertenbaker compares the back-stage dynamics of theatrical production to those of a republic. Through recognizing the need to sacrifice certain personal desires for the good of the "general will," through learning to cooperate in a joint-effort project and see ourselves as part of a social unit, we may stave off the threat of isolation and alienation so often remarked upon in (post)modern circles, creating instead real and surrogate families through patience, love, and trust.

Finally, this chapter suggests that drama facilitates experiments that cannot be conducted in a laboratory, thereby challenging cognitive scientists to consider the arts as essential companion-fields in the theorizing of human embodied cognition. The evidence presented in this chapter, including the testimonies of life-term prisoners who staged Our Country's Good in 1989, suggests forcefully that participation in dramatic production can instigate profound physical, emotional, intellectual, and spiritual transformation, affecting both individuals and their community at large.

Chapter 4

"A Spiritual Dance:" Moisés Kaufman's *33 Variations*

When this play's protagonist, Dr. Katherine Brandt, discovers she has an incurable disease, the rapid deterioration of her health and the inescapable demands thrust upon her by her physical disintegration, force her to inhabit the body she hitherto almost ignored. The radical cognitive shift that occurs when she becomes conscious of herself as embodied, just at the inception of that body's dissolution, precipitates an existential reconfiguration. Just as Shakespeare, in "Sonnet 18," hopes his poem will provide his beloved with immortality; just as Stoppard's Joyce claims his work will "double that immortality" (Chapter 2) so, in *33 Variations*, both the characters of Ludwig van Beethoven and Katherine achieve immortality through their respective works. However, I suggest that Kaufman's attitude to the necessarily finite nature of our existence also elucidates a condition Martin Heidegger terms "Being-toward-death."

As filtered through the productive dialogue between Romanticism and Existentialism suggested by the play, I propose that learning to trust the body, and learning from that body, does not cease when that body begins to fail. Quite the contrary. The deconstruction of the body may facilitate a reconstruction of the self; giving birth to a new subject position that can produce knowledge of a kind that could not, perhaps, be tapped by the healthy agent. Katherine's response to physical therapy prompts an analysis of the bodily effects of touch and their contribution to trust. And, finally, this chapter also considers spirituality in relation to the embodied emotion Jonathan Haidt terms "elevation."

This book begins by considering Shakespeare's demand that we awake our faith in the power of bodies in drama; it ends with Kaufman's suggestion that not only is the body not antithetical to spirituality, it may be its very source. The information provided by our feeling, communicating, meaning-making bodies permeates all existential domains. This information is never static or stable; it is always contingent, always evolving and changing. But learning to attune ourselves to this constant stream of information does not merely extend the scope of epistemological inquiry, it constitutes a necessary foundation for such inquiry and, by extension, forms the evidential basis from which we may evaluate whether or not to trust.

Chapter 1

"It Is Required You Do Awake Your Faith": Learning to Trust the Body through Performing *The Winter's Tale*[1]

> *"Alack, for lesser knowledge! How accursed*
> *In being so blest!"*
>
> (The Winter's Tale II.i.38–9)

> *"The drama of the human condition comes solely from conscious-*
> *ness…because it concerns knowledge obtained in a bargain that none of*
> *us struck: the cost of a better existence is the loss of innocence about that*
> *very existence. […] But drama is not necessarily tragedy."*
>
> (Damasio 1999: 316)

Skepticism is part and parcel of "a bargain none of us struck." There is no denying that human knowledge is limited, that there seem to be multiple, co-existing truths, and that these truths are also often in conflict.[2] However, we are not necessarily, therefore, forced to resign ourselves to radical relativism. Richard Rorty, for instance, claims that binary oppositions are misleading and that, accordingly, the values of true and false are only a "supposed antithesis" (Rorty 1984: 5). Paradoxically, he explains, the two sides depend on one another, define one another, and are in fact inextricably linked by a gradient that progresses from one to the other and does not allow for a clear-cut distinction.[3] But while Rorty sees in this predicament a basis for philosophic pragmatism that suspects all meanings and truths, the same concept of gradience has also been used to defuse the supposed threat of skepticism. Stanley Cavell and Ellen Spolsky both suggest that, despite lacking guarantees for absolute truth, humans still possess means of determining a gradient of truths that ranges from less probable, plausible, apt, or useful to those that are more so. Cavell claims, "it is possible to live an intelligent, satisfying, and even moral life with the mental equipment which is our inheritance" and "recover...from the tragically debilitating skepticism that rejects 'good enough' knowledge in a vain struggle for an impossible ideal" (Spolsky 2001b: 44–45).[4] Spolsky goes further, asserting that perfection is not only unattainable but that longing for it is counterproductive:

> Precisely because the human species and its ways of knowing evolved by the accumulation of random mutations in interactions with changing environments rather than genetically engineered for the task of knowing, it is not at all surprising that they are unstable. [...] It is just this instability, however, that provides the possibility for advantageous flexibility. People, their ways of knowing, and their languages are *responsive* (a word without the negative connotation of *unreliable* or *unstable*), that is, adaptable within a changing environment. [...]The evolutionary success of the species would actually be compromised by an entirely rigid, that is, dependable, representational system. (Spolsky 2001b: 52)

Both Spolsky and Cavell have studied *The Winter's Tale* as encouraging prudent skepticism, an intelligent questioning that counterweighs blind faith, dogmatism, and tyranny, while at the same time resisting the destructive lure of abandoned or unqualified skepticism. The play demonstrates that unqualified skepticism leads to self-betrayal: the destruction of both family and kingdom, but that it is a matter of wisdom and measure to understand that skepticism of the prudent kind is not only reasonable but productive.

In this chapter I consider the play's progression in terms of a stand against radical skepticism, which urges its viewers to place their trust in a creative form of faith expounded below. I argue here that, in the first half of *The Winter's Tale*, Shakespeare demonstrates the potentially paralyzing effects of doubt. However, in the second half of the play, he suggests how this paralysis may be countered by attunement to the instinctive human propensity to trust. Trust, as argued above and throughout this book, arises from *embodied* experience and, crucially, from our ability to use that experience in order to understand others. Through its metadramatic ingenuity, which stimulates resonance between living bodies on stage and in the audience, the combined effect of the thematic, structural, and performative aspects of *The Winter's Tale* prove not only the possibility but also the benefits of reconstituting trust in the body and the knowledge it provides.

I. The Malady of Reason[5]

At the beginning of *The Winter's Tale*, King Leontes suspects his wife, Queen Hermione, of conducting an illicit affair with his best friend Polixenes, King of Bohemia. Although Leontes's friends and advisors try to persuade him that his mistrust is unwarranted, Leontes's jealous rage cannot be checked. He humiliates Hermione in public and sends her to prison, paying no heed to the Oracle of Delphi who states clearly that Hermione is chaste. In prison, Hermione gives birth to a daughter. Paulina, Hermione's friend, brings Leontes the baby, hoping it will soften his heart. However, assuming the baby is the fruit of adultery, Leontes orders it to be left on a desert shore. Hermione is reported to die in prison and Prince Mamillius, Hermione and Leontes's heir, dies of grief at the news of his mother's death. Leontes, bereft of wife and son, realizes he was both mistaken and disproportionately cruel, but believes it is too late to save his family. In Act IV, we discover that Antigonus, directed by the king to dispose of the baby princess, leaves her in a basket on the seashore of Bohemia. Hermione then appears to him in a dream—or perhaps a vision that prepares us for her later exhibition of supernatural powers, depending on one's interpretation—and tells him to call the child Perdita, meaning "lost." Antigonus is then eaten by a bear. Perdita is, however, found by shepherds and raised in pastoral bliss according to the conventions of the green world. At the age of sixteen, Perdita elopes with her love, Prince Florizel. On reaching Sicily she meets Leontes and discovers her true ancestry. The oracle's prophecy is fulfilled.

In *Pandosto*, the prose-romance from which Shakespeare borrowed the plot for *The Winter's Tale*, King Leontes's suspicion of his wife's infidelity is raised by somewhat misleading appearances.[6] In *The Winter's Tale*, however, Leontes's suspicion is presented not only as wholly unprompted but—as other characters in the play immediately concur—the product of "diseased opinion" (I.ii.297). Leontes's diseased opinion rapidly develops into a jealous rage of such intensity that he seems mad. His madness is clearly not a justifiable response to any observation of his wife's behavior as Leontes himself first thinks, nor is it an explosion of (sexual) jealousy as his subjects first think. It is an "infection of [the] *brains*" (I.ii.144, my emphasis). This infection, as Cavell has argued, results from an unexpected and overwhelming exposure to radical skepticism (Cavell 1987: 15). The certainty of uncertainty threatens to destabilize his faculties to the point of insanity.

The Winter's Tale is often assumed to present an allegory of human folly, rashness, and violence, and to propagate belief in divine mercy,

achieved through Perdita-Nature and Hermione-Grace, the curative forces that ultimately right human wrongs.[7] And yet, the play
does not seem to rest upon a confident belief that divine mercy can
be trusted to wholly compensate for human mistakes. Shakespeare's
was a time of profound religious controversy and of renewed study
of ancient skeptical texts. The atmosphere of insecurity and doubt
regarding the very foundations of belief is reflected in the ways in
which *The Winter's Tale* dramatizes, again and again, just how difficult it is for humans to obtain secure knowledge. Firsthand experience of an event, although it seems direct, still fails to guarantee
infallible apprehension. Leontes's efforts to find unequivocal visible
evidence that his son is his (the nose, the shape of the head) are to no
avail because his confidence in appearances has been shaken. Leontes
gradually understands that two of his primary informing sources, the
modalities of hearing and seeing, are dangerously unreliable. The
third gentleman's bewilderment in Act V is expressed in the confusing possibility that "that which you hear you'll swear you see, there
is such unity in the proofs" (V.ii.32–3). But language proves no less
susceptible to confused misapprehension: although the words of the
oracle seem clear and explicit—"Hermione is chaste, Polixenes blame-
less, Camillo a true subject, Leontes a jealous tyrant" (III.ii.130)—
they are insufficient to persuade Leontes of his mistaken suspicions.

When the full force of the realization that meaning is uncertain
dawns upon the consciousness of King Leontes, disillusionment,
anxiety, and inordinate self-pity develop into anger, and soon after
into the abuse of others. When Leontes cries "All's true that is
mistrusted" (II.i.47) he reveals a desperation for an inverse truth-
guarantee. When he asks, "Is whispering nothing?" (I.ii.184) he is
confident that he knows it is not. He reasons that *if* all the signs of
his wife's adultery are nothing, *then* "the world and all that's in't is
nothing" (I.ii.293). However vehemently denied, the conditionality
of his hypothesis—the inescapable uncertainty that accompanies the
eternal open-endedness of signs and their interpretation—forms the
vortex of his crisis. Like Posthumus at a similar moment in *Cymbeline*,
Leontes convinces himself that his jealousy is justified as a means of
evading the alternative interpretation, which is that he cannot know.
Clearly, then, Leontes's madness is the expression of a crisis of faith:
he is propelled into a dark abyss from which it appears that the entire
world is unstable. The helplessness he feels colors the movement of
the tragic first half of the play, in which Leontes exaggerates the
imagined betrayal of his trust to a level that requires his conceptual
extinction of the whole world. His delight that he is blessed in his

"just censure" and "true opinion" becomes in the very next line a
dire realization that he is "accursed / In being so blest!" (II.i.37–9).
His knowledge seems to him "venom" (II.i.41).

It must be emphasized that Leontes is not driven to distraction by
any outside force or person. His mistaken mistrust and his ensuing
crisis are not caught like a virus from without, or inflicted upon him
by external forces such as destiny or divinity. Leontes's crisis necessarily indicates a form of personal choice—a response to the challenge
of doubt that misfires. He deliberately goes "angling" for evidence
(I.ii.180), encouraging Polixenes and Hermione to dispose themselves
to their "own bents," declining to join them when invited to do so,
and then determining their actions as proof of his cuckoldry (I.ii.191).
His interpretation of their actions is determined by his preconceived
suspicions. Because Leontes (like Othello) feels overwhelmed by his
powerful emotions of jealousy and anger, he mistrusts these emotions, hoping instead that reason will provide him with an anchor
for truth. However, as the play demonstrates, his decision to limit
his understanding to that which can be logically deduced through
strict reasoning leads him to form skewed notions. As the neurologist
Antonio Damasio avers, reason enables us to reflect upon and control
our emotions yet, since reason itself relies on emotion, its controlling
capacity is sometimes very limited (Damasio 1999: 58). Accordingly,
once Lenotes's reason is tainted by suspicion, it colors all he sees, rendering him entirely unreasonable. No "evidence" of any sort is admit-
ted as sufficient to preclude the possibility that he is being duped.

Psychologist Jonathan Haidt explains that this trajectory is predetermined by our cognitive architecture. The controlled system of
conscious thought allows people to "think about long-term goals
and thereby escape the tyranny of the here-and-now, the automatic
trigger of temptation" (Haidt 2006:16). But most brain activities are
automatic, and the automatic system was shaped by natural selection
to trigger quick and reliable action; it includes parts of the brain that
make us feel pleasure and pain (such as the orbitofronal cortex) and
those that trigger survival-related motivation (such as the hypothalamus). "The automatic system has its finger on the dopamine release
button [the neurotransmitter that allows us to enjoy pleasure]. The
controlled system may moderate behavior or calculate consequences,
but it does not initiate or cause behavior and is better seen as an advisor" (2006: 17). In other words, Leontes's extreme state of anxiety
prevents him from thinking rationally.

Shakespeare's portrayal of Leontes's behavior matches Cavell's assertion that "failure of knowledge is in fact a failure of acknowledgement,

the result of which is not an ignorance but an ignoring, not an opposable doubt but an unappeasable denial, a willful uncertainty that constitutes annihilation" (1987: 206).

Seen from this angle, it becomes apparent that for Leontes to suspect Hermione of adultery with Polixenes, he must ignore his long-term love relations with her and his long-term friendship with Polixenes; he must mistrust their history of virtuous, loyal, and loving behavior toward him; deny the affections they still express towards him, and instead imagine an intricate web of lies and deception. Logically, of course, this is not wholly impossible. As Leontes himself is quick to acknowledge, "There have been [...] cuckolds ere now" (I.ii.190). But Leontes's suspicion of Hermione—like Othello's suspicion of Desdemona—results from a blinkered reliance upon the possibilities afforded by logic that effaces all evidence to the contrary. Leontes's doubt arises from an internally generated, willful solipsism: he has chosen to shut himself off to questioning and knowing and, instead, to "believe [his] own suspicion" (III.ii.151). Ironically, relying upon faith alone, in this context, leads to false-belief and prevents Leontes from assessing the situation in an emotionally intelligent way. As Varela, Thompson, and Rosch have warned, "to deny the truth of our own experience in the scientific study of ourselves is not only unsatisfactory; it is to render the scientific study of ourselves without a subject matter" (Varela, Thompson, and Rosch 1991: 13–14).

What viable alternative process for decision-making does Shakespeare then propose? First, he dramatizes the benefits of alternative forms of knowing through his treatment of Leontes's greatest critics. For instance, Camillo defends the queen with an unflinching certainty that "recalls a medieval and chivalric sense of loyalty grounded in tradition and decorum rather than logic and intellect" (Landau 2003: 33). This axiomatic, unconditional faith is also extended by Paulina, who does not rely on the physical resemblances between Leontes and his daughter (to which she calls the king's attention), nor upon analytical refutations of the king's suspicions, but intuitively sides with her mistress, drawing her certainty from prior knowledge of Hermione's character. Systematically denying the evidence provided by the body, in favor of knowledge reached through reasoning alone, is highly dangerous, as Leontes's crisis of faith demonstrates. However, Spolsky reminds us that while the human brain has evolved a modular system, which can cause confusion and frustration because it allows for information obtained by separate modules to conflict, it is still, on balance, advantageous (Spolsky 1993: 5). Through memories, analogies, and inferences we are able to fill some of the gaps between dissonant kinds of knowledge categories, enabling problem solving, adaptability, creativity, and progress. Thus, instead of longing for unequivocal singularity, we benefit from a flexible attitude. In deciding upon our interpretation of our environment, and our responses to that interpretation, we are not determining what is true but only what is appropriate or useful at a particular point in time.

In precisely this manner, through taking into consideration the specificities of Hermione's character, personal history, and cultural background, and through allowing their intuitive interpretation of her conduct to inform their opinions, both Camillo and Paulina avoid the mistakes Leontes makes. Leontes's terror of insecurity leads him to seek ever more tyrannical means of enforcing stability. Soon his desire to halt the potential for proliferation of meaning is extended to encompass proliferation of his own bloodline. In his frenzied state, he refuses to acknowledge his own daughter and, instead, commands her death. This is the darkest point in the play's representation of Leontes's skeptical crisis. Its destructive energy is so great that it contributes to the death of his only son, Mamillius.

In the second half of the play, we learn that the best control against error—and against endlessly self-perpetuating doubt—is faith. However, faith does not equal unquestioning adherence to higher powers (whether fate, God, tradition, the law, or any others), nor is it presented as an escapist abdication of responsibility for assessing one's environment. Moreover, faith is not positioned as antithetical to reason. The terms "faith" and "trust" are used here somewhat interchangeably. This is because Shakespeare's use of the term "faith" does not indicate the truth of a particular system of religious beliefs but, rather, expresses confidence in the possibility of achieving satisfying knowledge and of fostering trust-relations among people. In line with Henderson and Horgan's definition of faith as grounded in a mutually beneficial "mix of strategies [...] jointly providing multiple modes of epistemic access" that complement and compensate for one another (2000: 123), faith in *The Winter's Tale* is a form of informed and conscious choice that mitigates doubt, suspicion, and hatred.

II. The Pastoral Cure

How are we to come by the collaborative knowledge that generates faith? One way is through learning from the long tradition of pastoral art and literature. Spolsky asserts that the function of the pastoral genre is to "correct an imbalance between an overdeveloped mental and an impoverished sensual life" (2001a: 17). As she points out, the conventions of the genre dictate that the hero(ine) spend a curative period in nature in order to "leave behind (temporarily) just the sophistication the high culture valued, and to abandon abstract knowledge in search of the satisfaction of learning that feels good, like a sunny day, good food, and sex without guilt" (2001a: 17). The hero(ine) then returns to city society, where his or her real destiny is to be fulfilled. This period away has provided the hero(ine) with a knowledge of nature and self, through channels that are either unavailable or shunned in the world of the city, where the values are tilted towards those of the mind.

In keeping with this convention, it is in retirement, far away from the court, that the characters of *The Winter's Tale* are brought in contact with the natural stimuli that encourage trust in embodied receptiveness. Perdita is brought up in bucolic Bohemia; Hermione takes refuge at Paulina's residence.[8] However, if we seek a pastoral interpretation for *The Winter's Tale* as a whole, we discover a problem: Leontes never actually leaves court. Martha Ronk offers a psychological interpretation of the play, by which the whole Bohemian interlude (Act IV) is a dream or a metaphorical representation of Leontes's private journey to peace; a visible dramatization of his invisible "internal struggle" (Ronk 1990: 56). Ought we then suppose that Leontes's sixteen years of self-flagellation and repentance served as his pastoral retreat? Can nature be so easily substituted? It is one thing to claim that this period serves as a time of punishment so that he may emerge worthy to win back his wife and daughter; it is less convincing to claim that Leontes has thereby learned the invaluable lessons that the body (and the pastoral genre) teach.

A different interpretation is offered by Valerie Traub, who argues that Leontes is driven mad by the fear of his wife's potential for erotic betrayal; that is, not by skepticism in general but by a specifically gendered and misogynistic anxiety. Therefore, she reasons, Leontes must show devotion to his dead wife and be delivered from the exigencies of female erotic life before he can re-enter marriage with any degree of psychic comfort. Meanwhile, Hermione's sexuality—"too hot, too hot!"(I.ii.108)—must be metaphorically contained and physically disarmed. Her silence towards Leontes in the last act of the play, according to Traub, bespeaks her submissiveness.

However, Traub's reading, focusing so forcefully on women's subjugation, fails to take into account the generic choice of the playwright. She claims Hermione is presented as a chaste statue in order to lessen the threat of her sexuality, but sexuality is one of the embodied sources of knowledge that the pastoral genre encourages us to admit as valid and valuable. If Traub's interpretation is accepted, and it may be said to complement New Historicist claims for the Early Modern theater's dynamics of containment, then it renders Act V a canceling out of Act IV; both Hermione and Perdita return to court, not to supplement its lacks but to be contained and nullified by it. This implies, furthermore, that the lesson Leontes has learned is that he may successfully dominate women and suppress both his own and his wife's sexual desires. Are we then to deduce that Shakespeare chose the pastoral genre only to discredit its power?

As I read it, the pastoral teaches how we may mitigate skepticism through trust. Leontes does not leave the court, but he learns the value of embodied receptiveness and effective communication through those he casts out: Hermione and Perdita. Hermione represents love, trust and loyalty. Moreover, her sensuality is not rejected as a form of wantonness but is recognized as a creative force. Her silence at the end of the play is, according to this reading, not a sign of submission but of triumph and regeneration. This interpretation is consistent with the advice that Cleomenes gives Leontes before Hermione returns: "Do as the heavens have done, forget your evil; / With them, forgive yourself" (V.i.5–6). Neither Hermione's nor heaven's forgiveness can substitute for self-forgiveness; Leontes cannot be fully cured until he forgives himself. This is not only to forego the weddedness to nothing (the skeptical abyss), nor merely a re-marriage to love (Hermione) but also a profound reconfiguration of his identity: the acceptance of an imperfect self. In the final scene of the play, it becomes apparent that the protagonists are not merely individual characters but characteristics. Leontes's reason and doubt are united with Perdita's natural-knowing, and Hermione's love and forgiveness. The (re)unification of this family also symbolises the necessary mixture of qualities required for a balanced life.

Like Leontes, many of Shakespeare's contemporaries sought to fend off the threat of uncertainty through increased religious dogmatism and scientific positivism. In contrast, many poets and artists became increasingly suspicious of rigidity, celebrated instead the mysterious opacity of poetry (Orgel 1991: 437). In *The Winter's Tale*, Shakespeare expresses his discomfort with inflexibility by ignoring strict generic categorization and continually undercutting his own symbolism. Just as, according to pastoral conventions, city life and its sophistication are supplemented by the wisdom of nature, so in this play the conventions of the pastoral genre are themselves supplemented by those of romance. A conventional romance structure typically unfolds a tale in which the hero is limited in his ability to control his destiny, teaching humility. In *The Winter's Tale*, the hero's destiny is subject to a strange mixture of Christian and pagan divine powers, borrowing both from ancient mythology and the traditions of medieval miracle plays. This lends a theological character to the romance action and subjugates it to the tragicomic message.

Tragicomedy was famously dubbed "mongrel" by Sir Philip Sidney (1595) because it merges the sublime with the ridiculous, joy with sadness, an awareness of darkness with optimism. Similarly, Shakespeare seems to insist, life cannot be neatly categorized into generic units. Illogicality, discontinuity, coincidence, frustration, and surprise abound in life. Therefore, it is fitting to represent these in art by using a "mixed mode" of expression.[9] As Stephen Greenblatt observes, this mixed mode "exposes the instability and uncertainty of human judgment...It forces the reader to call into the open and examine consciously those standards by which he judges experience. [...] For the mixed mode, to resolve is to lie" (Greenblatt 1973: 351, 355).

Shakespeare's mixed mode complements Henderson and Horgan's claim that epistemic competence is best achieved through "hybrid processes" (2000: 130). Similarly, it seems analogous in many ways to the cognitive theories outlines in the introduction to this book, particularly the paradigm of reciprocal connectivity: "a hybrid mechanism, combining innate perceptual-motor coupling with acquired context-action associations" (Borenstein and Ruppina 2005: 232). "Hybrid" does not imply random, motley patchwork, but sophisticated, adaptive responsiveness. *The Winter's Tale* convinces us that "hybrid" is not only "good enough" but the best option we could choose. Through adopting a stance of informed flexibility and searching for truth while agreeing to modify our conclusions as we proceed, we allow ourselves to develop a skill that is of greater potential value to us than the search for definitive absolutes. If we choose to develop our *receptiveness to possibilities*, to perceive ourselves as ever-open to suggestion, and ever-adapting, we do not thereby lose some innate centralized truth that requires vigilant protection but, rather, locate ourselves within a field of interactive communication: a constant movement that feeds off, and back into, our personal and collective environments. This dynamic, I contend, has already been suggested by the coalition of functions that constitute our cognitive spectrum. When we consider philosophy through the paradigm suggested by biology, we discover that we do not have to feel alienated or isolated, but, rather, we can feel part of an interactive process of exchange, which extends and refines our potential for reaching truths.

IV. A (Winter's) Tale of Embodiment

In an attempt to gather satisfying knowledge, humans not only deploy hybrid forms of knowledge acquisition, which allow for a broad base for potential understanding, but have also developed tools for bypassing biological limitations and extending cognitive abilities. One of these tools is the telling of stories. As Suzanne Keen notes, we are "story-sharing creatures" (Keen 2006: 209). The status of tales and their relation to truth(s) are at the very heart of *The Winter's Tale*. The phrase "an old tale" is repeated twice in Act V (ii. 30, 65) echoing the title of the play. The second gentleman says: "This news, which is called true, is so like an old tale that the verity of it is in strong suspicion" (V.ii.30–1). Walter S. H. Lim maintains that Shakespeare foregrounds classical mythology in *The Winter's Tale* not simply to facilitate the demands of plot but also to "accentuate his interest in the status of different generic forms: the ballad, the ghost story, classical myth, and even the Bible itself" (Lim 2001: 317). The focus of interest becomes not theology but the representational space of literary production, the Bible becoming just one, rather than *the*, (literary) text.

Cavell holds that the activity of telling denotes "reconceiving, reconstituting knowledge, along with the world" (1987: 204). To speak, he argues, "is to say what counts" (205). Telling, therefore, implies accounting for what matters. In tales, because the value of events is worked out in the telling, the act becomes one of *re*counting. Cavell notices that Hermione's somewhat erotic pleasure in having tales told in her ear (II.ii.34 "Come on then, and give't me in mine ear") must be known to her husband and may therefore be one of the causes of his exaggerated suspicion of her whispering with Polixenes and then with Mamillius. Retelling tales in this context implies the sensuality of proliferation and fertility.[10]

Shakespeare, as a dramatist, takes this a step further. As argued above, his use of the pastoral genre emphasizes the importance of combining intellectual assessment with receptiveness to physical and emotional signals; his extension of the pastoral genre into a mixed-mode of generic experimentation allows for multiple registers of meaning that instantiate his suspicion of rigidity. His decision to convert a prose-romance into drama, I further suggest, allows him to combine and maximize many bodily, sensory stimulants to add experiential force to the tale itself. The most fantastical events in *The Winter's Tale*—the king's daughter is found, his courtier is eaten by a bear,[11] and the queen is miraculously resurrected (either from death or retirement, depending on one's interpretation)—are all expressed as events that have to be seen to be believed, since experience of them "lames report," "undoes description," and lies beyond the capacity of "ballad-makers...to express" (V.ii.26–7). The scene in which Perdita is "found" is *reported*, while the scene in which Hermione is "found"—lacking the naturalistic explanations of her daughter's fate—is *shown* in the most spectacular, theatrical manner. In the final minutes of the play performance overrides words, as Shakespeare follows Aristotle's advice that "as far as possible, [the poet should] also bring [his plot] to completion with gestures" (*Poetics* I.xvii 4.3.2). After her "resurrection," Hermione is expressly asked by Paulina not to spoil the atmosphere by troubling their joys with "like relation" (V.iii.130). Thus, Hermione's silence may, after all, signal neither submission (Traub 1992), nor love (Cavell 1987), but rather the power of theatricality. Didactic explanations would spoil the emotional impact of this scene. Silence allows the departing theater audience to leave with an unmediated tableau imprinted in their minds. Though discussion will surely follow, the last image of the performance is that of a gesture.

V. A Tale Performed: Theatrical Spectacle as Revelation

The silent gesture with which Shakespeare ends the play is carefully prepared by the entire final act. In Act V of *The Winte's Tale*, after sixteen years of self-flagellation, abstinence, and regret, King Leontes is united with his daughter Perdita. Then Paulina, Hermione's friend and the wife of Antigonus (who was eaten by a bear), invites them to her gallery to view a statue of their late wife and mother Queen Hermione. When the statue is unveiled, the likeness is so striking that the characters are moved to tears. Then a miracle takes place and the statue comes to life. Much has been written about this scene. Is Hermione really brought back from the dead? Was this ever really a statue, and did it then turn into flesh? In which case, is this black magic or divine intervention? Perhaps it is a sign of Shakespeare's Catholic inclinations and a propagation of the power of images in the face of Protestant iconoclasm? By this point in the play "such a deal of wonder is broken out" (V.ii.25) that the theater audience is made to feel uncertain whether to believe what it is *told* by Paulina and how to interpret what it *sees*.

The only explanation we receive for Hermione's revival is Paulina's command: "It is required / You do awake your faith" (V.iii.95). What, then, does this faith entail? In Act I Leontes believes Hermione has been unfaithful, even though he has not directly witnessed her infidelity. Nothing that comes by way of council can convince him of the falsity of that belief, and his obdurate blindness foregrounds the gulf separating conviction from truth. "Translated into the discourse of religious conviction, belief in things unseen does not necessarily add up to possessing the truth" (Lim 2001: 321). Instead, if Paulina's conduct in the play is to demonstrate good faith, we can only infer that this entails neither unconditional submission nor non-interventionist passivity that trusts in divine direction. Whether by hiding the queen, pretending she is dead, castigating Leontes, ensuring he does not remarry or, finally, by orchestrating the (seemingly) miraculous resurrection of Hermione in Act V, Paulina's actions are instrumental in determining the outcome of the play. Paulina's kind of faith also deploys secrets and lies—withholding information and disseminating misinformation—in order to achieve its ends.[12]

By reminding us of the ease with which language can be deliberately manipulated to conceal knowledge, Shakespeare undermines the Protestant epistemological claim for "sola scriptura"—meaning that the words of the scriptures are enough to contain and explain all truths. This seems to reinforce the claims that the anti-rationalist implications of *The Winter's Tale* suggest an affinity with Counter-Reformation ideology and aesthetics (Landau 2003:30). Landau infers that Shakespeare is trying to impart the following message:

> only a regained sense of foundational faith, untarnished by a rationalist quest for religious knowledge and couched instead in the sensuousness of ceremony and ritual, only a recovery, in other words, of a residual sense of late-medieval and proto-Catholic religiosity, can afford English society to look beyond its traumatic present state of religious division and strife. (Landau 2003: 29)

The play does indeed seem to include "a veiled critique of Protestant religiosity" (2003: 30) as well as a wide range of possible political subtexts, but I contend that the crux of this critique is not a particular religious persuasion; rather, it is primarily dramatic.[13] Mystery, sensuousness, and ceremony are aspects of Catholic faith that the Protestants eschewed, and the concomitant suspicion of idols and images has been described as creating a hunger for spectacle (Spolsky 2001a). But the "resurrection" in *The Winter's Tale*, though it takes place in a chapel, is in fact a *staged performance*. A visual analogy is created between the pulpit and the stage, suggesting theatrical performance is a source of potential revelation. The fact that Paulina uses language in order to disguise, rather than to explain, emphasizes that her real efforts take place in the material world of *actions* and *interactions*.[14]

This explains Shakespeare's prioritizing of showing over telling. Instead of relying upon didactic, rationalist arguments (which may recall the kind of positivism he critiques)—he causes the audience to feel directly. As explained in the introduction to this book, our understanding of the potential meanings of actions is assisted by "motor equivalence."[15] In the process of simulation, one adopts another agent's perspective by "tracking or matching their states with resonant states of one's own" (Gallese and Goldman 1998: 493) creating a "correspondence" (497) that establishes a link "constituted by the *embodiment* of the intended goal, shared by the agent and the observer" (Gallese 2001: 36).[16] Precisely this level of embodied engagement is required in order to make sense of *The Winter's Tale*. The meaning of Hermione's statue can only be understood if audience members acknowledge their instinctive, *embodied* mechanisms of cognition. When Perdita wishes to kiss the hand of the statue, she is halted by Paulina who claims the colors are "not yet dry." In performance, Perdita is usually presented as believing this excuse, though viewers are more likely to understand that, since Hermione is real, kissing her hand would give away the mystery. By maintaining distance Paulina maintains doubt regarding the wonder of the statue. In contrast, however, the audience does not have to touch Hermione to *know* that she is real. Although performance greatly determines the extent to which the characters on stage appear to believe that a supernatural miracle is taking place, or suspect that some clever trickery is being practiced, the audience's experience of the discovery of the statue is an instantaneous Gestalt (comparable perhaps to the sudden shock Leontes experiences when confronted by the skeptical realization). The instant the statue is uncovered audiences know at once that *this is the queen*. Her living body is immediate testimony that she is the same Hermione of Act I. The audience are not fooled by Paulina's cover story.

Director Nicholas Hytner agrees that performance does away with many of the questions that seem unresolved in the text. Hytner writes that *The Winter's Tale* is made believable, and thence meaningful, through attention to the physicality of the characters. Noting

Mamillius's nose requires wiping (I.ii.121) and later that Hermione's skin has wrinkled (V.iii.28) emphasizes that *The Winter's Tale* is about "flesh-and-blood people" (Hytner 2002: 22), grounding this often fantastical tale in common human experience. Moreover, in every performance he has either directed or attended, no one in the audience ever doubts that Hermione is alive (Hytner 2002: 22). The playtext may encourage multiple interpretations but performance overrides texts. Even if the actor is very skilful, the audience knows, by virtue of having bodies themselves, that this is not a lifeless statue. Embodied receptiveness convinces us that the "tale" of Hermione-as-statue is wholly unbelievable. This is crucial. The presence of the queen's body on stage—the unequivocal realness of the flesh—sufficiently dispels doubt. The fact that in Shakespeare's day a boy would have performed the part of Hermione does not affect this argument, as it is the life of the *body* that gives away the lie. Clearly, Shakespeare trusted in his audience's embodied receptiveness.

Furthermore, the moment audiences understand that the statue is alive, they must reorganize the information of Acts III and IV in order to accommodate a new interpretation of the play's events that allows for Hermione having remained alive all this while. In determining this new, retroactive interpretation, I submit, we are not so much relying upon sophisticated theoretical or literary skills as upon the most primitive embodied mechanisms of simulation and motor equivalence. Thus we learn, in a very real sense, by *physically participating in observed action*. Naturally, Shakespeare knew nothing about neurobiology. But as a dramatist and an actor he was intuitively aware of, and glad to exploit, our innate attributes. Religious positivism suspects all spectral evidence and subordinates all human knowledge to the unfathomable will of an omnipotent God. Shakespeare's faith suggests that, within the realm of human existence and inter-personal interaction, our knowledge, confidence and potential for communication depend upon trusting not in higher powers but in our own bodies and the knowledge they provide.

What then is the point of this trickery? Celebrating drama. When the statue is revealed, spectators not only know the queen is alive, they also empathize with the performer's physical challenge of remaining motionless for so long. Even if we are seated in a large theater and cannot see that she cannot refrain from blinking, we immediately understand why Leontes thinks "the fixture of her eye has motion in't" (V.iii.66). Thus, the audience is invited to engage with the emotions of the major characters but also, at the same time, to engage with the physicality of performance. Accordingly, though the audience is wholly aware that this is a performer pretending to be a queen, pretending to be a statue—an entirely artificial situation—the success of the scene nevertheless depends upon basic embodied resonance. Further still, the advocacy of skilled interaction in *The Winter's Tale* is best conveyed in performance because it is in performance that the audience experiences the extent to which moments of silence connote action. Hermione dominates the final scene by virtue of her positioning (most probably elevated, perhaps even on a pedestal). She need not speak to command the attention of those on stage, as it is for the purpose of seeing her that they have come to Paulina's gallery, while the other characters must rely more heavily on words to be noticed. Though the "resurrection" of Hermione may perhaps be designed to celebrate the miraculous power of (divine) forgiveness, it is first and foremost a show of impressive ingenuity: of Paulina and Hermione's masterful stage directing. Once we understand this, we are in the position to perceive another dimension of irony in Leontes's remark that, through the statue, "we are mocked with art" (V.iii.66). Above all else, this meta-theatrical scene demonstrates the creative power of theatrical performance.[17]

In performance we are also more likely to note that the few words Hermione does utter in this scene are spoken to Perdita:

> ...I
> Knowing by Paulina that the oracle
> Gave hope thou wast in being, have preserved
> Myself to see the issue. (V.iii.127)

The second syllable of the word "Myself" is stressed at the beginning of the line and is usually stressed by the actor in performance. This indicates that it is neither a miracle nor Paulina that is responsible for Hermione's return but, rather, Hermione herself. Additionally, her speech indicates that she has preserved herself not for Leontes but for her daughter and her grandchildren—for the prospect of issue that Leontes had once tried to obliterate. In retrospect, the second gentleman recalls that Paulina "hath privately, twice or thrice a day, ever since the death of Hermione, visited that removed house" (V.ii.114–115) in which Hermione is finally revealed. This too suggests that Hermione has chosen to remain in hiding until the oracle's prophecy should come true and her daughter be found. When Leontes cries that he has "in vain said many / A prayer upon her grave" (V.iii.140–141), he indicates that he now understands she was never dead but only "thought dead" (V.iii.140). And his final remark is even more telling:

> …Good Paulina,
> Lead us from hence, where we may leisurely
> Each one demand and answer to his *part*
> *Performed* in this wide gap of time since first
> We were dissevered. Hastily lead away. (V.iii.152–155 my emphasis)

The words "part" and "performed" are placed in the closing lines of the play to accentuate their vital role in the play's resolution.

The Winter's Tale calls for skepticism to be pondered as a solution rather than a problem, an opening of multiple possibilities rather than a threat to knowledge. Human knowledge is always provisional, always suspect; human apprehension and interpretation are often unreliable. But, as Leontes discovers, shared understanding can often be reached if we acknowledge the evidence provided by the body. Neither philosophy, nor religion, nor educated guess work suffice to explain this scene. The status of miracles is never fully clarified. Instead, we are commanded to awake our faith (V.iii.95). This faith, I have suggested here, is not a form of unquestioning trust in providence or in divinity, for Shakespeare delights in the possibility that trusting in miracles entails believing events that are in fact displays of artistic creativity. Faith implies trusting in human resourcefulness and in acknowledging the powerful potentials of kinetic knowledge, intuition, memory, inference, imagination, experience, and creativity—all of which should be the means of attaining knowledge that is "good enough" to form the basis of healthy trust-relations with our fellow human beings. It is trust in bodily knowledge that grounds the leap of faith we are required to make at the end of the play. Hermione's living body communicates directly with our own.

Preoccupation with the representational and philosophical implications of a play, especially its truth-value and its implication in dominant discursive structures is undoubtedly valuable. But, as Mary Thomas Crane has rightly complained, it may obscure what performance makes clear (Crane 2001: 173). Performance is a material process, by which actors and audience participate in the process of making meaning. This includes both the intellectual exercise of unpacking the play's meanings, and the pre-conscious embodied participation in observed action that stimulates both neural and motor circuits. The optimistic ending of *The Winter's Tale* is not, then, a contrived forgetting of uncomfortable events and their inherent violence. By witnessing murder desired and forestalled on stage, audiences experience identification with violent impulses and then both the cathartic release and of those impulses and the containment of their negative effects. If we may learn from a play without having to make the mistakes it *re*counts, without suffering ourselves, without inflicting terrible damage upon others, and without waiting sixteen years, then Shakespeare has succeeded in demonstrating the genuinely miraculous power of art and convincing the audience that performance, far from being malicious falsehood, is both enthralling and restorative. The knowledge that emerges from performing *The Winter's Tale* is invaluable: in order to overcome the paralyzing effects of radical skepticism and its potentially tragic implications, and in order to convert this knowledge into a productive force, Leontes—and the audience— must "awake [our] faith:" faith in the generative and curative powers of performance on the stage as in our lives.

Chapter 2

"A Doubling of Immortality:" Cognitive Inter(con)textuality and Tom Stoppard's *Travesties*

. . . for one man calleth wisdom, *what another calleth* fear; *and one* cruelty, *what another* justice; *one* prodigality, *what another* magnanimity; *and one* gravity, *what another* stupidity. . .

(Hobbes 1651 I.iv.24: 27)

For the game of creation [. . .] a sacred "Yes" is needed
(Nietzsche 1891 Part I Speech 1: 139)[1]

I. *Freeplay* or Freefall? The Risks of Postmodern Skepticism

Skepticism can function as a safety net: protection against believing that which may be untrue. But Skepticism has its own inherent dangers, as evinced in Chapter 1 of this book. Many Postmodern theorists have embraced a particularly relativistic form of skepticism, which they inherited, by degrees, from Reformation thinkers.[2] This is one of the reasons for which this book opens with a chapter on Shakespearean drama.

From the moment Protestantism advocated an unmediated relationship between man and God, it laid the foundations for conceptions of truth and value to become personalized. It is not by chance that the ancient Greek skeptical texts were rediscovered and received renewed attention in the Early Modern period. By the time of the Restoration, the climate was ripe for Thomas Hobbes to be able to publish his view that the knowledge we derive from our senses is only of singular, particular things. This provides no grounds for believing in any absolute or universal Truths. Universals are, according to Hobbes, products or functions of the human mind, of thought processes mediated through language. Thus, when we speak, which is a useful and necessary tool for communication, we are only naming our thoughts and not any objective reality. Ascertaining truths is a logical procedure, an exercise that considers linguistic constructions, not ontology. "For *true* and *false* are attributes of speech, not of things. And where speech is not there is neither *truth* nor *falsehood*" (1651 I.iv 11 23). In this respect, Hobbes is the forefather of the radical relativists of the twentieth century, who admit to no truth but linguistic conventions— Lyotard's "phrase-regimes."

The democratization of truth has proven at once liberating and threatening. If taken to the relativistic extreme, by which reality becomes an array of (subjective) options that are equally viable, all anchors for reality are undermined. When Walter Pater asserted in *Plato and Platonism* (1893) that "truth itself is but a possibility, realizable not as a general conclusion, but rather as the elusive effect of a particular personal experience" (Pater 157), he was celebrating the freedom afforded to the aesthetic critic by acknowledging reality to be the product of the impressions of the individual. Truth had become both subjective and multiple.[3] But Pater was not overly concerned with society or morality. Nietzsche, on the other hand, acknowledged that "in us the will to truth becomes conscious of itself as a *problem*" (1887 III 27: 597). Nietzsche declared that the pre-requisite for intellectual rigour, and moral living, is that it should be possible to pass definite judgments without excess doubt concerning values. However, while this renders it necessary that something should be assumed to be true, it does not make any belief actually True: "what is needed is that something must be held to be true—not that something is true" (1901 III iv 507).[4]

Truth, then, is something for which we may strive, but there is no one or real Truth. In fact, according to Nietzsche, art, in which "the lie is sanctified" and "the will to deception has a good conscience" (1887 III 25: 589) best expresses the will to life and facilitates self-affirmation, faith, cheerfulness (the gay science) and also self-improvement.[5] He famously announced that he distrusts "all systematisers" as "the will to a system shows lack of honesty" (1889 I, maxim 26: 470). But honesty does not entail anarchism or nihilism; it entails the courage to be continually in an active, creative process of re-evaluating ones values. As opposed to the tendency to simply "worship the question mark itself as God" (1887 III 25: 592), Nietzsche called for a courageous commitment to "Saying Yes to life" (1889 "What I Owe the Ancients" v: 562).

Distrust of *Truth* is often extended to encompass all notions of *truths* and has gradually led to the prevalent Postmodern trend Susan Haack terms the "fashionable disenchantment with truth" (Haack 1999: 14). This trend undermines the very pursuit of knowledge since, as Haack laments, unless one's conclusions are true they cannot be said to contribute to knowledge, only to "purported knowledge." The result is a "gradual erosion of intellectual integrity" (ibid). Postmodernism replaced the concept of truth with the concept of interpretation—"a field of infinite substitutions" (Derrida 1972: 260)—thereby engendering an epistemological crisis. For, while Barthes celebrated *jouissance* and Derrida delighted in the *freeplay* of language games, the effect of the insistence on multiplicity, fragmentation and instability has often been bewilderment,[6] producing a particular breed of skepticism which posits that truth is, more often than not, controlled by (invisible) power sources.

From Foucault and Lacan until recently, agency, power and its manipulation have been the focal issues of Postmodern criticism. This has enabled various critical communities to reassess and redefine moral standards, the culturally acceptable and the literarily valuable. Although serving to empower political minorities, these routes of inquiry have also often substituted Nietzschean or Derridian playfulness with suspicion, encouraging sectarian mistrust among people and peoples. Esther Beth Sullivan describes this predicament as "enlightened paralysis," the state of having internalized the understanding that ideological oppression is not forced upon us from without but manufactured from within by the invisible processes of cultural and political osmosis, and yet of lacking a viable way to generate action (Sullivan 1993: 149). The image of ourselves as isolated individuals, as necessarily contesting subject positions, also erodes commitment to community and so, eventually, to ethical and moral responsibility. We become isolated, impenetrable.

If we do not acknowledge our influence upon others and act accordingly, we effectively abandon accountability for our actions.[7] Christopher Norris argues that in the 1990s, Postmodern relativism amounted to "a wholesale collapse of moral and intellectual nerve, a line of least resistance that effectively recycled the "end-of-ideology" rhetoric current in the late 1950s" (Norris 1993:1).[8] By substituting any notions of ontological grounding with a "hyperreality" of language games, we are not merely effacing solidarity, responsibility for many social ills and the people who suffer by them, but our own potential for social criticism, for informed critique, for thought at all. Believing only in relativistic, textualist positions and discourse games compromises the very possibility of seeking to redress social injustices. If one's critique is to hold any water, one must argue for some level of knowable reality, an experience-based understanding that can be shared among different people, even if their values or opinions differ.

Tom Stoppard's play *Travesties* creates an elaborate and impressive affirmation of Nietzsche's celebration of life and Barthes's call for *jouissance*. By presenting the absurdities of life, Stoppard is not expressing Pyrrhonist resignation that chooses to laugh at—rather than despair of—an incomprehensible world.[9] *Travesties* is set during the heyday of the Modernist era but considers that era from a Postmodern perspective. By juxtaposing these two artistic epochs Stoppard is able to recall the positive elements of the Modernist project, while combating the less desirable effects it has had in Postmodern theory. The play portrays a world in which meaning can not only be attained but effectively communicated.[10] *Travesties* suggests that art can express forms of truth in which we may justifiably trust.

Stoppard accomplishes this by leading his audiences to partake in a tightly orchestrated journey of "reason in madness." *Travesties* is infused with such an air of insanity that it is often believed to celebrate disorientation, nonsense and even chaos.[11] However, the play should not be understood to endorse all that it explores. Stoppard's mastery of Dada ideology does not indicate that he necessarily adheres to it, nor does it align him with the Absurdist traditions of Dada, Surrealism and some French Existentialism.[12] Tyrus Miller has pointed out that "a historically layered context of *theories*" may be "the predominant factor" of avant-garde art-works. The other "necessary element" is that audiences must learn how to "construe, recognize and apply heuristic tools" in order to grasp the specific problems that the works pose, inextricably linking theory and art (Miller 1999: 557, 574). Close examination of *Travesties* reveals that Stoppard stretches Dada to its limits, thereby demonstrating its shortcomings. As he himself has claimed: "If a play has an easily comprehensible meaning, it's a failure" (Stoppard to Maves 1977; Delaney 1994: 100).

In *Travesties*, the character of Carr refers to Dada as a "historical halfway house" between Futurism and Surrealism, between "before the-war-to-end-all-wars years and between-the-wars years" (*Travesties* 8). Dada was an attempt to effect, through disorder and disorientation, a drastic dislocation of the artworld. Through destroying all existing parameters, Dada hoped to open the way to new ones. Similarly, as

Stoppard explains in his stage directions, the narrative of *Travesties*, like a toy train, often "jumps the rails and has to be restarted at the point where it goes wild" (*Travesties* 11). However, unlike Dada art, *Travesties* not only gets "restarted," it also leads in a specific direction; the chaos of Stoppard's stage is immaculately structured. As Steven Connor writes, "the principle of disarrangement and incompleteness" that seems to govern the play, in fact creates coherence where dislocation is most expected, and relies on a theatrical style that demands "perfect precision" (Connor 1996: 111, 113). Stoppard has specified not only the words the characters speak but the relative volume of enunciation. He specifies props, costumes, sound and light effects, seeking to control every element of the performance-experience in order to ensure that its "wildness" does not merely confuse but, rather, re-configures. There is no fixed, true reality in this play, but when "reality" slips into fantasy, Stoppard is careful to signpost the rollercoaster ride. An example of this is the scene in which Cecily and Carr first meet in the library, that lapses into a progressively raunchy, striptease-cabaret.[13] Stoppard's directions stipulate that, the moment we enter into Carr's imagined fantasy, colored lighting plays over Cecily's body, while the song "The Stripper" plays in the background. Audiences immediately perceive they are witnessing a reverie.

II. The Non-Characters

Travesties was initially inspired by the historical coincidence that brought three world-transforming figures to Zurich at the same pivotal period in history—The First World War. James Joyce (1882–1941) the author of the archetypal Modernist text, *Ulysses*; Lenin (1870–1924) founder of Bolshevik Communism and legendary leader of Soviet Russia; and Tristan Tzara (1896–1963) the infamous Romanian-born French Dadaist. These three were all living in Switzerland during the war. However, the meeting between them is a figment of Stoppard's imagination. Thus, from the start, Stoppard blurs the distinction between fact and fiction, history and art. Moreover, the imagined encounters between the three historical titans are "recalled" by Henry Carr, an English civil servant, who was also living in Zurich at the time. The historical Carr did, in reality, meet Joyce but neither Lenin nor Tzara. Joyce's subsequent antipathy to Carr is expressed in *Ulysses*, where Carr figures as an irritating minor character.

The historical James Joyce put on a production of Oscar Wilde's *The Importance of Being Earnest* in Zurich in 1918, in which Carr acted the part of Algernon. This fact is used by Stoppard as a spring-board for his play. In *The Critic As Artist*, Wilde argues that master-ful cultural analysts, as exemplified by Ruskin in *Modern Painters* and Pater in *Studies in the History of the Renaissance*, make the artworks they discuss "more wonderful" through the creative impressionism of their responses (1891: 1694). Masters, suggests Wilde, do not merely describe the artwork, but treat the work of art "as a starting point for a new creation." This new creation is not an imitation of the original, nor is it confined to the intention of the original artist (which may or may not be known). "For when the work is finished it has, as it were, an independent life of its own, and may deliver a message far other than that which was put into its lips to say" (Wilde 1891: 1695). This seems to me to be an accurate description of Stoppard's own inter-textual cross-fertilizing technique. In *Travesties,* Stoppard functions both as masterful critic (of a spectrum of Modernist revolutions, both aesthetic and political) and as (Postmodern) artist.

Stoppard appropriates Wilde's comedy of errors plot and quick-witted style, along with the characters of Cecily, Gwendolyn, and Bennett-Lane the manservant. However, he deliberately confuses and inverts their identities, so that these characters do not mirror but, rather, subvert Wilde's characters.[14] Wilde's and Stoppard's word games call meaning into question, disturbing any illusion of a singu-lar relation between word and referent, signifier and signified; while double-entendres, perceived or overlooked by the characters, sug-gest that reality is determined by verbal skill. As Wilde's Gwendolyn so eloquently phrases it: "In matters of grave importance, style not sincerity is the vital thing" (*Earnest* III: 353). Stoppard also adopts Wilde's classic comic ending, the matching up of two couples for mar-riage. In *The Importance of Being Earnest*, this generic convention travesties the illusion of order in the face of the crumbling of values and social structures of *fin de siecle* England. In *Travesties*, the same comic ending travesties the illusion of order in 1917, during the Great War and the Russian Revolution.

Travesties also challenges the conventions of the memory play. The events of the play are presented through the prism of Old Carr's fail-ing/selective/creative memory, where historical events, frustrated ambitions, "senile reminiscence" and "digression" *(Travesties* 6) are "reshuffled like a pack of picture cards" *(Travesties* 35) with fictional texts. Wilde's Cecily maintains that memory "usually chronicles the things that have never happened, and couldn't possibly have hap-pened" (*Earnest* II: 333) and this is precisely what Carr's memory does in *Travesties*. For the most part, as Brian Richardson notes,

Carr's "misrememberings are grotesque deformations (or rather, anti-memories) of the events they purport to recall" (Richardson 2001: 683). At other times, they are impossibly accurate. For instance, he "recalls" scenes that he did not witness, such as Lenin speaking in the library, which, moreover, takes place in Russian, a language he cannot understand. Thus, as Stoppard himself notes, the audience is under the control of an erratic and unreliable man of "various prejudices and delusions" (*Travesties* 11).

Moreover, *The Importance of Being Earnest* is not *Travesties*' only intertext. Barthes argues that texts are comprised entirely of fragments of linguistic matter quoted from anonymous sources, a collage of pieces of language brought into spatial proximity. As Owen Miller explains, this proximity invites the reader to "create some sort of patterning by forcing them to discharge some of their interrelational energy" (Miller 1985: 24). *Travesties* is an explosion of such "interrelational energy." It includes references, (mis)quotations, puns, and parodies of a myriad of literary texts including Tennyson, Kipling, Gilbert (and Sullivan), nursery rhymes and T. S. Eliot, to mention but a few. Toby Zinman has called *Travesties* a "spectacular (and auricular) homage/burlesque of western culture's most dazzling era, from Romanticism through High Modernism" (Zinman 2001: 124).

Stoppard's ultra-educated literary acrobatics and phenomenal cultural repertoire serve to ensure his audience a night of both funny and surprising entertainment. But this is by no means the sole intention of the playwright. As Stoppard explains: *Travesties* is an attempt to "marry the play of ideas to comedy or farce" (Stoppard to Hudson et al.; Delaney 1994: 59). Comedy is a means by which he enables the conflicting ideologies of his characters to be presented, examined, parodied and ultimately judged. It is their ideas—political, aesthetic, and social—that stand at the center of the play. The plot structure, style, and even characterization are subordinated to this purpose.

Stoppard has expressly asserted that, "What interests me is getting a cliché and then betraying it" (Stoppard to Bradshaw; Delaney 1994: 96). In *Travesties*, each character possesses enough defining characteristics to be recognized as Joyce, Lenin, or Tzara, without being developed into an intricate personality. Stoppard does not merely show disregard for emotional engagement between characters and audience, he deliberately forestalls it. This technique serves to direct the audience's attention towards the ideational debates dramatized in the play. In turn, these debates efface the humanitarian concerns of the play's historical setting, seemingly doing away with morality. Thus, the play may be supposed to undermine both emotional identification and moral values and has indeed elicited responses, such as Ileana Orlich's, who describes Stoppard's characters as funny yet extremely sinister (Orlich 2004: 372). The audience is presented with cultural icons, chosen as characters for their uniqueness, and is encouraged to wonder at their originality, their genius, their perversity, but not their common humanity. In fact, their egocentrism repels in a form of counter-identification.

But audiences must not suppose this to express fidelity to Brecht or Becket. The apparent disdain for empathy and the desire to dislocate, distance, even alienate the audience, are all part of the Modernist project, which this play openly questions. From the late nineteenth century Symbolist movement, through to the early twentieth century Modernists and Existentialists, identification and emotional contagion were sacrificed for a distilled, stylized, aesthetic, and ideational experience. However, just as he does by replicating Dada techniques in order to show its limited range, so too Stoppard skilfully deploys counter-identification in order to discredit it.[15]

Orlich, for instance, holds that failing to maximize identification with the characters renders *Travesties* forever an intellectual exercise, never quite permeating or affecting the audience. But this view rests on a misunderstanding of the nature of empathy. First, as Damasio (1999) and LeDoux (1998) concur: thoughts and emotions cannot be separated; thinking involves feeling. Second, though personal dispositions to empathy vary, empathy itself, as mentioned in the introduction to this book, is not synonymous with conscious emotional identification, more accurately related to sympathy. Empathy functions on multiple levels, many of them pre-linguistic and preconscious. Third, "empathy for fictional characters appears to require only minimal elements of identity, situation, and feeling" and such empathy is extended to characters that are "not necessarily complex or realistic" (Keen 2006: 214).

As discussion of the pastoral genre in *The Winter's Tale* showed in Chapter 1, interpretation is more likely to be satisfying if it takes account of the choices made by the playwright. The counter-identification effected by *Travesties* must be viewed as an experiment Stoppard himself conducts by choice. Plays such as *The Real Thing* or *Indian Ink* show that Stoppard is wholly capable of creating emotionally engaging characters in realistic plays. *Travesties*, however, plays a different game. Finally, this is a play—a dramatic performance—and no one is more aware than the playwright of the fact that all ideational, conversational, intertextual, and linguistic games are subordinated in performance to the strategies of its presentation on stage—and the (in)voluntary embodied participation of the audience. The notion of a farcical play of ideas incorporates the concept of game, but also of dramatic performance. As explained above, Stoppard's dramatic precision encompasses every aspect of performance; every detail in the play is designed for particular effect. Shakespeare teaches us that dramatic performance serves revelation; Stoppard skilfully co-opts the embodied potential of dramatic performance in other but equally effective ways.

Thus, *Travesties*' audience is aware that the characters they are watching are partly based on reality, but neither historically accurate nor realistic; that they are riotously funny, but certainly not merely farcical; that they are related to, represented as, and reconfigured by at least one of Wilde's characters, but this serves to complicate, rather than explain their meaning and significance; and that they also express contradictory opinions that relate in multiple ways to other ideas, texts and histories which cannot possibly all be grasped during performance. However, Stoppard does not allow the viewer to feel lost in a maze. The viewer's attention is carefully directed by *actions performed on stage*, which provide visual focus and clarity to the verbal turmoil. For instance, whether or not a viewer managed to follow all the different strands of the argument between Tzara and Joyce in Act II (discussed at greater length below), it becomes clear that while Tzara can only read from the pieces of paper he has cut up, Joyce can turn them into carnations and white rabbits (*Travesties* 44). It is clear he has the upper hand, not merely because he is arrogant and aggressive (which he is) but because he is truly more sophisticated, more talented, and in possession of singular finesse. Thus Stoppard elicits greater respect and admiration for Joyce and positions his opinions as weightier and more convincing.

Other scenes are demystified without the use of words and without the need for identification. In the very first moments of the play, which take place in the library, Stoppard's stage directions stipulate that production should ensure the audience *observes* Gwendolyn receiving a folder from Joyce, and CECILY receiving an identical folder from Lenin. These folders, assumed to contain manuscripts, are brightly-colored. Each girl has cause to put down her folder for a moment, and each girl then picks up the wrong folder (*Travesties* 2). This technique—as old as pantomime itself—relies on the audience's most basic space-time understanding. Our mirror-matching neural circuits fire on observing an action we perceive as intentional; our object-recollection mechanisms convince us of the women's false-belief mistake; the eye-catching exterior of the files ensures we both notice and recall them. Not a word is exchanged, yet empathic engagement is secured. Similarly, the confusing lapses of reason and memory that Carr experiences throughout his narrative are regularly marked by the resounding amplification of a cuckoo clock (*Travesties* 11). Apart from referring significantly to time in Switzerland, the effect is remarkably powerful in performance, driving home the audience's suspicion of Carr's sanity.

III. The Creative Cure: Cognitive Inter(con)textuality

The characters, perhaps better described as caricatures of the historical personages they represent, passionately believe in incommensurable worldviews. Each in turn declares his manifesto without seeking or accomplishing any measure of effective dialogue with his interlocutors. The only positive connections made between characters during the play are of a romantic nature. While these connections can be termed "embodied," since they arise from physical attraction, they are entirely divorced from the political and artistic revolutions that form the subject matter of most other interpersonal exchanges in the play. Thus, it may appear that Stoppard is reinstating the old binary distinction between intellectual and sensual understanding, the latter mocking and undermining the former. As one of the notes that Joyce pulls out of his pockets at the very beginning of the play reads: "Entweder transubstantiality, oder consubstantiality, but in no way substantiality. . ." (*Travesties* 3). Apart from referring to the Catholic vs. Lutheran conceptions of the Eucharist, raising metaphysical questions regarding miracles and magic, two elements that define the core of his art-philosophy, this scrap also indicates a rejection of substance. Does Stoppard's play do the same?

No. Carr describes Joyce as exhibiting "a monkish unconcern for worldly and bodily comforts."[16] In this sense—if Carr's description is to be believed, which it need not be—Joyce represents an anti-embodiment argument. But, as already noted above, Stoppard uses embodied performance tactics to elevate Joyce above the other characters. Not only is the multiplicity of opinions built into the style of the play-text, but the very competition between speakers is often decided by the volume of Joyce's voice, which quite literally drowns out Tzara's (*Travesties* 4).

Unlike *The Winter's Tale* (Chapter 1) and *Our Country's Good* (Chapter 3), *Travesties* does not set out to encourage trust. Other plays by Stoppard could be argued to accomplish this task more successfully.[17] However, *Travesties* has been chosen for this chapter because it is a self-conscious experiment, and suggests a powerful antidote to the relativistic skepticism of Postmodernity. Stoppard's answer to "enlightened paralysis" (Sullivan 1993: 149) lies in a celebration of multiplicity, which is nevertheless contained and thereby prevented from collapsing into infinite regression.

This is achieved through an interlacing of disciplines I term *Cognitive Inter(con)textuality*, which is anchored in a process of supplementation. The supplement is both an addition to an already whole entity and also a necessary completion of an insufficient entity. Thus, it describes the creative process by which brain, body, and world collaborate in producing meaning. As demonstrated in the following pages, supplementation also expresses the relation between intertext and focus text: the text is in itself complete, yet if it may also be enriched by the intertext, then it was, by implication, also somehow incomplete. Supplementation also describes the very structure of language, which is in turn determined by the architecture of the human brain. In other words, Stoppard acknowledges the processes by which human brains create meaning, and suggests how we make take advantage—rather than despair—of them.

Texts, intertexts and their potential for meaning proliferation are at the core of *Travesties*. At the opening of Act I, Tzara, Joyce and Lenin are all reading and writing at the Zurich library.[18] Joyce is writing his novel by rewriting Homer's *Odyssey* with the assistance of Gwendolyn and the Dublin Street Directory for 1904 (*Travesties* 26). Tzara is creating poetry by cutting up Shakespeare's sonnets, placing them in a hat and then rearranging the words in random order. Lenin is rewriting Plato, Marx, and soon the entire future of his country, while Stoppard rewrites them all in the context of Wilde's play and through the medium of Carr's memory.

(Re)writing, (re)contextualizing, (re)defining, (re)evaluating, using past texts and ideas to forge new ones, and using critique and parody to ground innovation, are not strictly literary activities. Cognitive scientists and linguistic theorists agree that this is how most human thought is produced. Damasio defines consciousness in terms of the relations between organisms and objects, between the entity understood as self and external entities (Damasio 1999: 20, 133). Knowledge necessitates assessment of the relations between at least two separate facts/objects/entities. Lakoff and Johnson assert that objects do not have inherent qualities so much as "interactional properties": they are understood relative to one another (1980: 163). Stoppard's image of Zurich during World War I, packed with "spurious spies peeping at police spies spying on spies eyeing counter-spies" *(Travesties* 12), reflects the activity of politicians and artists reflecting upon one another, shedding light on each others' words and worlds. But it also dramatizes the necessary link between them: the "interrelational energy" that emanates from their interaction.

Moreover, as argued in the previous chapter, body and mind, brain and environment, co-opt and supplement one another in a *creative process*. By processing information we necessarily generate meaning(s). These meanings may or may not occur to other people observing the same input. Understanding is not simply a case of eliciting ready-made meaning; it is greatly determined by subjective experience, individual talent for interpretation and imaginative scope. Consider, for instance, that vision is concentrated in the visual cortex but, so far, thirty different areas have been identified within this cortex. Form, color, depth, and movement, are each processed by a separate region (Livingston and Hubel 1988). This saves a great deal of time, as these regions can all function simultaneously. It also allows for cross-referential safeguarding: as the regions are relatively independent of one another, so that one can be fooled by an optical illusion, while the other corrects the misapprehension (Eagleman 2001). Most pertinent to the present argument, the visual system is itself interpretive. The information coming in through the eyes is not projected into the brain as is. Instead, it is disassembled and re-configured by the brain, so that our mental image of the world is constructed by a creative mind. This creative (re)construction relies heavily on memory. We automatically fill in the gaps of missing details by drawing upon past experiences: previously established CDZs. "Change blindness" experiments, for instance, show how attention-directed perception is (Silverman and Mack 2006; Auvray et al. 2007).

Humans regularly invert, ignore, distort, connect, supplement and even invent in order to create an image that seems to us at any given time acceptable, logical, accurate. Vision does not produce a mirror-image but, rather, a creative synthesis performed by the brain. This relatively new information adds weight to Stanley Fish's assertion that "we are never not in the act of interpreting, there is no possibility of reaching a level of meaning beyond or below interpretation" (1980: 631). Stated thus, it appears that we are all, to a degree, artists. By thinking, using language and trying to understand one another, we are engaging in the inferential processes States calls "infra-association" (2001: 112): exercising our capacity for creating meaning.

Of the different means at our disposal for articulating meaning, language is often the default choice. Linguistic competence is one of the subjects the characters of *Travesties* discuss. The seventeenth-century dream of finding/coining a precise word for every object and phenomenon in the world has not only proved impossible to achieve, it has been shown to be undesirable. The fact that language works by "capturing *approximate* meanings" whose degrees of similarity or difference "express our experience sufficiently well and sufficiently often to be useful" (Arbib and Hesse 1986: 152, 155), enables words to apply in different contexts, as circumstances require, assuming slightly altered semantic signification in the process, while still being understood. The fact that we bring words we already know to bear on new contexts allows language to continually regenerate and develop. Fixity would cause stagnation and prevent the kind of fluidity necessary to meet the challenges of a changing world, while flexibility encourages the creativity and adaptability the world requires.[19] As Spolsky explains, "the very flexibility that destabilizes meaning is not only good enough, it is responsible for our success, such as it has been, in building and revising human cultures" (Spolsky 2002: 43).

In *Travesties*, Lenin and Carr profess to believe in realism, logic, purpose, cause, and order. Their preferred view of language is therefore literal, assuming that a word can stand for a single well-defined fact or idea (Carr *Travesties* 21). Tzara, on the other hand, considers any form of order or causality illusory. Tzara champions abstraction, nonsense, chaos. The fact that Carr and Lenin are associated with an old fashioned and rigid approach to language illustrates their desire to control and contain the fertility of language, and reflects their authoritarian preferences. However, Tzara's advocacy of non-meaning is not presented as an advisable alternative. His claim that "nowadays, an artist is someone who makes art mean the things he does" functions as a parody of Humpty Dumpty's equally childish insistence that "when *I* use a word . . . it means just what I choose it to mean—neither more nor less . . . The questions is . . . which is to be master—that's all" (Carroll 1872: 197).[20] Stoppard acknowledges the Derridaen freeplay of language as an infinitely useful tool for creativity but, at the same time, he also acknowledges that language and meaning are subject to external limits.

Travesties demonstrates that language is not singular, but neither is it wholly arbitrary. This assertion has since been developed by Owen Miller, who holds that each (inter)textual fragment refers at once to intra, inter and extra textual connections. Thus, intertextuality rejoices in multiplicity, addressing itself to a plurality of concepts yet, at the same time, creates a unifying force by grouping them together in a broad relationality. Despite its inevitable plurality, signification is

not deemed an entirely unmanageable "promiscuity" of infinite proliferation (Miller 1985: 25). Similarly, in *Travesties*, the bewildering
lack of an anchoring referent implied by polysemy is grounded. Both
Lenin and Carr's strict literalness and Tzara's "promiscuous" proliferation of infinite (non)meanings are shown to fail.

Stanley Fish argues that "all sentences are ambiguous . . . No degree
of explicitness will be sufficient to disambiguate" (Fish 1980: 636).
Nonetheless, he explains, not all interpretations are equally viable.
Any utterance is always "naturally" understood in relation to the *context* in which it was uttered. There are "no inherent constraints on the
meaning a sentence may have," yet "agreement is not only possible
but commonplace" by virtue of the "shared background" which per-
mits the interlocutors to understand one another (644). Utterances
are communications. We are called upon to *interpret* these *communications* in a *context*, which necessarily delimits the range of possible
meanings the communication may have.[21]

Stoppard demonstrates just this when he overrides both Carr-
Lenin's and Tzara's approaches to language. He does this, significantly, in reference to a text, Joyce's *Ulysses*, in which Joyce uses
fragments of speech, stream-of-consciousness and other seemingly
impermeable linguistic devices reminiscent of Tzara's cut-ups, in
order to encourage the reader to piece together a semi-coherent tale
that *does* make sense. When Tzara woos Gwendolyn by cutting up
Shakespeare's "Sonnet 18," we discover that, as Gwendolyn pulls the
words out of his hat, they do not amount to nonsense but, rather,
remain a love poem—different and more vulgar, but still a love poem.
It appears that even when the professed intention of the speaker is
to create non-meaning, human cognition cannot fail to tie words
together and create meaning.[22] This process of imaginative creation
has been demonstrated by clinical research: "when events demand
explanation but lack visible causes, *causes must be invented*" (Premack
and Premack 1995: 207, my italics).[23]

A pattern thus emerges: singular true/false binary categories are
insufficient to describe meaning, yet there are nevertheless determining contexts that prevent total anarchy. I argued in Chapter 1 that our
response to skepticism is largely a matter of choice. Similarly, meaning construction is a form of personal choice. Every action we witness, every statement we (over)hear, invites us to embark on a process
of interpretation. This process is necessarily one of personal creativity. And yet, as Miller explains, we cannot justifiably interpret in any
manner we please: we are limited by the options that the text/utter-
ance/action and its context lend. Thus, as Miller argues, meaning

must be viewed as "an implication rather than a presupposition;" it is "imposed to some degree (like an implication) by certain constraints of the text" (1985: 34, 35).

I hope that by now my term "cognitive inter(con)textuality" is becoming clear. The linguistic expression of meaning is both inspired and determined by context, which is analogous to the activity of supplementing through intertextuality. This activity is naturally facilitated by the cognitive processes that human brains have evolved that, as discussed in the introduction to this book, exhibit a preference for relationality. The means by which we supplement the apparent lack in the text mirrors the impetus for flexibility and creativity in art, just as it is the core impetus for change and advancement in life. Language is innately intertextual and, by extension, all meaning-construction is intertextual: that is the way our brains function. Stoppard claims that his plays do not forward a single, committed or clear statement but, rather, offer "a series of conflicting statements made by conflicting characters, and they tend to play a sort of infinite leap-frog" (Stoppard to Hudson et al.; Delaney 58). This is precisely how our modular cognitive system operates. In turn, *Travesties* evokes a wide range of socio-political, philosophical, and aesthetic debates, creating textual interfaces that are generated in relation to one another. It is a highly sophisticated example of the Postmodern endorsement of semiotic polyvalence. However, as I have been indicating, not all options are given equal emphasis or equal standing. Not all interpretations are endorsed.

IV. Mimesis, (Postmodern) Parody and Doubling Immortality

The genre of parody is a particularly useful tool for illustrating an *inter(con)textual* approach to literature. Of all artistic genres, parody relies most heavily on intertextuality, since its very purpose is to engage with other texts.[24] However, parody must also restrain proliferation of meaning. If an intertextual reference is detectable only in exceptional contextual circumstances, the reference must be relegated to the realm of aleatory, private discourse (Miller 1985: 35). Such parody is very rare in the Postmodern age because, as Linda Hutcheon explains, the Postmodern audience is recognized as disunified, multiple audiences with varied fields of reference that do not always overlap with those of the author. The pervasive Postmodern "lack of faith in systems requiring extrinsic validation" is expressed in art forms that "incorporate critical commentary within their own structures in a kind of self-legitimizing short circuit of the normal critical dialogue" (Hutcheon 1985: 1).[25] Thus, the Postmodern composition—musical, visual, or literary—is relied upon to reveal the methods by which it can/ought to be comprehended.[26] Hutcheon claims further that (Post)modern culture has developed a particular fascination with systems that "refer to themselves in an unending mirroring process" (1985:1). Instead of seeing parody as plagiarism, nostalgic imitation of past models, or a form of ridicule (though it can be those too), Postmodern parody presents "a stylistic confrontation, a modern recoding which establishes difference at the heart of similarity" (Hutcheon 8). By recontextualizing the text(s) it engages, parody performs a creative resemanticization.

The degree to which *Travesties* confirms Hutcheon's theory is striking. It also provides a means of coming to terms with the texts of the past, recalling in many ways "the giant age before the flood:" the Classical and Renaissance attitudes to cultural patrimony, which pre-date what Harold Bloom has called the "anxiety-of-influence" (Bloom 1997: 11).[27] Past giants and their works are simultaneously revered, commemorated, and ridiculed, the ultimate effect being the establishment of a bridge between past and present.

In addition to its parodic mirroring-techniques, *Travesties* addresses the playful creativity of the "unending mirroring process" of culture (Hutcheon 1) through one of its central substructures. Ever since Plato first spoke of the stage as a mirror, fiction in general and drama in particular have been considered in terms of *mimesis*—imitation or reflection.[28] In *Travesties*, Lenin lives on *Spiegelglasse Srasse*, or *Mirror Street*, and it is not by chance that "across the way at Number One" (*Travesties* 8) stands the Meierei Bar of the Dada gang, placing revolutionary artists opposite the revolutionary politician. Howard D. Pearce has shown that Plato's underestimation of the (philosophical) potential of the arts is analogous to his misrepresentation of the potential of the mirror. "The mirror's versatility lies in perspectives. It is always in only one place, but from that vantage it can turn in all directions" (Pearce 1143). In accordance, *Travesties* reveals drama's capacity not merely to reflect but to refract, making the essence of *mimesis* plural; making art a form of creative supplementation.[29]

As discussed at length in my introduction to this book, mirror-matching seems to be "a basic organizational feature of the brain" (Gallese 2001: 46). Our ability to adapt and fit into our social environments is largely determined by our ability to understand the behavior of other individuals in each environment. This ability relies upon bodily mechanisms that match observed behaviour with the mechanisms of the observer. Gallese argues further that this dynamic also extends into "social cognition," implying that the "relational nature" (Gallese 2001: 39) of relationships is modelled upon our biological (infra)structures. Stoppard's play, in this light, becomes a challenging mirror image of our cognitive processes. *Travesties* deconstructs the distinctions between dream/reality, fact/fiction, stage/world, exposing these to be not clearly separable dichotomies but, rather, distinctions that set up reflections. Tzara's art-revolution and Lenin's world-revolution are not merely mutually antagonistic; they mirror one another, with all the complexity that implies, and are further fractured by Joyce who, significantly, lives on *Universitatstrasse* (*Travesties* 24) and Carr, who conflates all categories.

The insistence on plurality also informs the treatment of the categories of art and politics. Zurich during the Great War was, as Joyce explains, "the theatrical center of Europe," partly because it was politically neutral, like Joyce himself, partly because it served as a site for "the continuation of the war by other means" (*Travesties* 32). In fact, the political debate in the play is determined by each character's attitude to art. Stoppard's Joyce argues that the only meaning history can have is in "what survives as art" (*Travesties* 41). One would initially expect Tzara, who practices art for art's sake, to side with Joyce against Lenin the realist, but Tzara opposes Joyce. Kinereth Meyer has noted that, in the idea that Chance rules all, Tzara, like Lenin, "denies the authority of the individual artist," paradoxically revealing "an affinity with the stringent control of artistic expression imposed by dialectical materialism" (Meyer 110). This claim is extended by Orlich, who argues that Dada's belief that history advances through the clash of opposing forces and not through negotiation, shows a dedication to Marx's dialectical view of history (Orlich 376). The Dada aesthetic and the communist ideology are shown to agree in violently opposing the bourgeois establishment. Thus the seeming incommensurability of their positions is blurred.[30]

Stoppard clearly objects to Lenin's organized-State-art of practical utility, which conflates art and propaganda.[31] But neither does he take the side of the "bourgeois individualists" (*Travesties* 59) represented by Wilde and Tzara. Stoppard exposes the flaws in both ideologies: neither a stringent structuralism nor a completely unrestricted anarchism (or Derridian post-structuralism) will do. Lenin's polemic against individualist art is shown to stem from his recognition of its power to affect the emotions. Despite himself, he is moved by art, especially music (*Travesties* 62). On the other hand, the social chaos and moral abandon of Tzara's Dadaism is demolished. First of all, logically speaking, whether the causes of the war were noble patriotism and desire for freedom, or oil-seeking and money-grabbing (*Travesties* 22), there were still causes, direct and tangible. The war did not occur by chance. Second, Tzara may be rejecting traditional art forms but, like any good Modernist, he is seeking a privileged and elevated position for art within culture. Moreover, he may call for an anti-art of Chance but it is still art, an activity in which he engages with a level of passion that Joyce finds ridiculous (*Travesties* 41).

Stoppard's art-vision, having conflated and deflated both Tzara and Lenin, rests with Joyce. As Stoppard has explained in an interview:[32]

> Instinctively I am out of sympathy with Tzara and that kind of art, and I had to think very hard to give Tazra good arguments in the play. My prejudices were all on Joyce's side—I utterly believe in his speech at the end of act I on what an artist is . . . Joyce has the last word. I wanted him to murder Tzara and he does. (Stoppard to Wetzsteon 1975 :121)

This claim is instantiated in performance when, during their argument over these issues (mentioned briefly above), Joyce brushes off the scraps of paper left in his hat by Tzara when "writing a poem" for Gwendolyn. He places the cut-ups back into the same hat, but the effect is altogether different form that which Tzara was able to accomplish. In Joyce's possession, the hat produces a white carnation, which he then tosses at Tzara. Tzara cannot respond in kind, admitting Joyce's triumph to be an example of "enterprise and charm receiving their due" (*Travesties* 40). Tzara may be adventurous and creative enough to invent a new form of theory/art of nonsense, but it is Joyce who performs the magic tricks; it is Joyce who creates beauty (a flower) out of chaos. The debate with Tzara is concluded by Joyce pulling a white rabbit out of the same hat (*Travesties* 41).[33] In turn, Joyce's creative polysemy, contained by artistic form, becomes the model Stoppard himself adopts for his play.

And yet, Stoppard has no scruples about travestying Joyce, whose self-importance is far from endearing. Joyce is irreverently compared to an old matron, because initially mistaken for one by Carr, and consequently called Doris, Janice, Phyllis, Diedre, and Bridget (*Travesties* 32–4, 68) but rarely Joyce, and anything from a "prudish prudent man" to "a liar and a hypocrite, a tight-fisted, sponging, fornicating drunk" (*Travesties* 6–7).[34] Joyce's arrogance may be partly justified by writing a literary masterpiece, something that cannot be said of Tzara. On the other hand, Tzara's delight in the absurd and his playfully self-contradictory attitudes enact a kind of self-parody that mirrors the self-parody of Stoppard's play. Stoppard's play (like Wilde's) travesties earnestness.

Carr rages at the very idea of the artist as a special kind of human being,[35] but Tzara argues that even hunter-gatherer tribes had artists, "priest-guardian[s] of the magic that conjured the intelligence out of appetites." Without artists, he declares, humans would be no better than coffee-mills: "eat-grind-shit" (*Travesties* 29). Having said that, however, Tzara also revolts against Joyce's assumption of the role of "priest-guardian of the magic." He accuses Joyce of having turned art into a religion just at the time religion itself died. The time for subtlety and genius is over, he cries; in order to overturn all fallacious cultural moulds "we need vandals and desecrators, simple-minded demolition men" (*Travesties* 41). The accusation that the Modernists viewed themselves as the alternate priesthood is not unfounded.[36] But Joyce holds that the artist is a magician chiefly because he gratifies a basic human urge for immortality (*Travesties* 41).

According to Joyce, if there is any meaning in life "it is what survives as art," even in the "celebration of nonentities" (*Travesties* 41–2). By being travestied in *Ulysses* and then in *Travesties*, Carr is ultimately saved from obscurity. In reflecting upon the dead Joyce, both Carr and Stoppard affirm their existence. By travestying Joyce and *Ulysses*, through which, claims Carr, it became apparent that Joyce was in possession of "an amazing intellect bent on shaping itself into the permanent form of its own monument" (*Travesties* 6), Stoppard is also shaping his own "amazing intellect" into his own monument. If the *Odyssey* commemorates Troy and Odysseus, Joyce claims that his Dublin will "double that immortality" (*Travesties* 42). *Travesties* is the ultimate doubling of immortality, commemorating Wilde and his *Earnest*, Joyce and his *Ulysses*, Tzara, Lenin and Stoppard himself. As Shakespeare's "Sonnet 18" decrees before Tzara cuts it up:

> So long as men can breath and eyes can see
> So long lives this and this gives life to thee.

Travesties demonstrates that great art is far more than pulling random words out of a hat; it requires genius, inspiration and finesse. And the rest is magic. This claim abounds with optimism and defies paralyzing skeptical doubt and its self-indulgent earnestness.[37]

Moreover, *Travesties* performs—literarily and literally—a critical defiance (a deconstructive dynamic) which is simultaneously the institution of a viable alternative (a constructive dynamic). Jürgen Habermas lamented, in the early 1970s that Modernism's avant-garde was mistakenly believed to have been superseded and negated by Postmodernism, while it was in fact "an incomplete project" awaiting "fulfilment" (Habermas 1981: 137). *Travesties*, I suggest, constitutes just such fulfilment. Habermas believed that, by the 1970s, the aesthetic of the avant-garde had passed its *Jetztzeit*: it began to repeat itself, lose its edge, go out of fashion. Habermas blamed this on two factors: first, a general mistaking of the effects of capitalist-economic developments for effects of Modernist intellectual efforts and, second, the failure of the Dada-Surrealist revolution of art for art's sake. The reasons Habermas puts forward for this failure are identical to those Stoppard ridicules in *Travesties*. First, limiting art to the expression of the artist's subjectivity, detached it from all constraints, creates a schism between art and society (Habermas 1981: 133). Second, the attempt to explode *all* previous notions of art is too radical. In order for a new concept to be understood, it must be incorporated into previous conceptual patterns that provide a stable base for the new structure.[38] In other words, progress relies upon a communicative relationship between old and new. As Habermas explains: "Nothing remains from a desublimated meaning or a destructured form; an emancipatory effect does not follow." Total negation is useless, it is merely "terroristic" (Habermas 1981: 134). *Travesties*, written in 1974, both rejuvenates the avant-garde aesthetic just at the point Habermas marks its demise, and also confronts precisely the notions of credible, meaningful revolution (Lenin, Joyce) vs. mere terroristic destruction (Tzara). Stoppard's play creates an environment in which old and new not only co-exist but activate reciprocal relationships. Despite the apparent meaninglessness of the first scene's exchanges—and Stoppard is perfectly aware that the majority of his audience does not speak Russian, German, and French so that at least some of the dialogue and puns are necessarily lost upon them—every sentence does in fact yield intelligible meaning to an educated ear. Similarly, not everyone recognizes the innumerable literary echoes, (mis)quotations, and references, but these do exist.

Habermas further argues that Modernity "lives on the experience of rebelling against all that is normative. It is addicted to a fascination with that horror which accompanies the act of profaning, and yet is always in flight from the trivial results of profanation." These attitudes "find a common focus in a changed consciousness of time," a "cult of the new" that finds expression in exaltation of the present. Simultaneously, the value placed on the transitory, the elusive, and the ephemeral, "discloses a longing for an unidentified, immaculate and stable present" (128). *Travesties* celebrates dynamism while also evoking a nostalgic longing for stability. As Carr explains in the play, Switzerland's alluring charm lies in the "ostentatious punctuality of public clocks" that gives the place a "reassuring air of permanence" (*Travesties* 10). In the midst of a world war, revolution and uncertainty, the promise of a safe haven is irresistible. But, paradoxically, the people attracted to this haven are refugees, exiles, spies, anarchists, artists and radicals of all kinds (*Travesties* 45). It is as though the "miraculous neutrality of it, the non-combatant impartiality of it" (*Travesties* 8) acts as a vortex that sucks in radical non-conformists; as though its peace were analogous to Derrida's textual lack that requires supplementation. Political neutrality and its promise of permanence are revealed to be an incomplete condition, a gap. Artists are instinctively drawn to fill this gap with vibrant and volatile activity. However, *Travesties* arranges the congregation of artists and revolutionaries in Zurich during 1917, in an artistic composition that acts as a guarantor of permanence. Not the clocks of Switzerland but "what survives as art" will ensure immortality. However, even immortality will not be singular but, rather, double *(Travesties* 42).

V. Carr as Artist

Ironically, it is Carr who brings together all the different strands of the play and shows us how art and life intertwine. Carr's surprisingly creative use of memory becomes the very nucleus of art. Although Carr partakes of art by having acted in the play Joyce put on, he has failed to write a book (*Travesties* 22). And yet, *Travesties* is entirely Carr's creation, and it is so fanciful that one may wonder whether his imaginative skills were wasted. He apologizes that the encouragement of poetry writing was not the primary concern of the British consulate in Zurich in 1917, and lack of practice has diminished his flare (*Travesties* 6). But has it? In a way, Carr becomes an Everyman figure with whom the audience can identify; his artistry is just the kind of inferential processing, directed by individual preferences, biases, memories, and fantasies that each of us engages in daily.

Initially, sharing Lenin's distrust of modern art (*Travesties* 60), Carr announces that to be an artist at all is like living in Switzerland during a world war, but to actually be an artist in Zurich, in 1917, implies "a degree of self-absorption that would have glazed over the eyes of Narcissus" (*Travesties* 38).[39] He philosophizes that if one is not a revolutionary, one might as well be an artist; but if one cannot be an artist, one might as well be a revolutionary (*Travesties* 98–99). Pearce argues that while Lenin, Tzara, and Joyce are revolutionaries in their field, and counter-revolutionaries in the others' fields, fulfilling at least one of Carr's categories, Carr is just ineffectual and bitter. But this is not quite accurate. Despite the young Carr's refusal to play the game of linguistic multiplicity (shocked and confused by Tzara as much as Alice is by Humpty Dumpty) the old Carr's pseudo-literary description of Zurich is a sham of linguistic free-association, making the river "snot-green" by virtue of a Latin pun (mucus mutandis), but equally recalling Joyce's "grey sweet mother" and "snot-green sea" and Kipling's "great grey-green greasy Limpopo River" (Sammels 384–5).

Carr in fact exhibits surprising flexibility, wit, and charm. He is dragged into the freeplay of the world by the force of vanity (to perform before an audience the character of Algernon, for which he requires new clothes), then by the force of love (for which he assumes the character of Tristan in the library), and finally by the force of old age. In old age, he continually confuses himself with Algernon (almost never named but as "the other one") so that when he recalls buying the famous trousers that become such a point of contention between himself and Joyce, he is buying them both *as* and *for* Algernon: "the trousers, etcetera, purchased by me for my performance as Henry—or rather—*god dammit!*—the other one" (*Travesties* 43). This statement reveals a slippage between past and present, which could be a product of old age, or could have already occurred during 1917. It may reveal a repressed desire for Algernon's nonconformity or it may imply that the character of Henry Carr is nothing but show, a performance he plays to the world. Carr's over-identification with a fictional character is also a comment on the reality-fiction deconstruction at work in the play.

But Carr seems well aware, at least in old age, of the profits of the identity game. First, it won him a bride, for it is in disguise that he woos Cecily. Second, while frequently referring to the "truth" and the "facts" of the matters he discusses, Carr is not limited by fidelity to either and is fully aware of his tendency to get carried away: "take no notice, all come out in the wash, that's the art of it" (*Travesties* 7). Memory is a form of art. Indeed, it is in the face of Cecily's (accurate?) recollection of facts that his narrative rejects accuracy as deplorable pedantry. This suggests that either Carr was always far less pedantic than he appears in his own recollection/ (re) construction of his conversation with Tzara, or he has learned, having reached old age, the pleasure of creative use of language and history. This may be proof of having gained insight into the workings of the world, or may be a way of venting his frustration at having been the one who stayed, while others moved on. Such possibilities combine in any case to make a self-reflexive comment on Stoppard's drama, in which an actor plays Carr, who plays Algernon, who confuses seeming with being. But, more than anything, it expresses a vision of life-as-art.[40]

Intertextuality is not simply a critical approach to literature, but to life. Intertextuality provides a model for an interconnected world, which corroborates cognitive research that suggests we are biologically designed to perceive the world in terms of relational values. The fact that our mind is a modular mechanism led us to create language and art that are equally modular, relational, inter(con)textual. Philosophically, this realization provides a comfort to those depressed by the supposed loss of a center, and those bewildered by the Postmodern concept of freeplay. We are creative, responsive individuals who operate within multiple interpretational-communities, and our ability to understand, communicate, and even predict is, as Cavell reassures us, "good enough." Derrida calls for the Nietzschean "joyous affirmation . . . of the freeplay of the world" (Derrida 1970: 268)—which he recognizes as determining "*the noncenter as otherwise than as the loss of center*"— and Stoppard responds through with his own riotous freeplay: *Travesties*.

VI. From Writing to Performing

Travesties exhibits a preoccupation with writing, a motif already suggested by Wilde's *The Importance of Being Earnest*. Neil Sammels asserts that the "fundamental lesson" of Wilde's play is that "all writing is a lie we cannot do without" (Sammels 1986: 382).[41] Indeed, as both Cecily and Gwendolyn's diaries demonstrate, writing distorts facts and creates fantasy; it neither documents nor reveals truths. The most renowned example is Miss Prism's sentimental romance manuscript, which she mistakenly places in a pram instead of the baby Jack-Ernest, whom she leaves in a handbag at Waterloo station. This confusion between fact and fiction is echoed in *Travesties* when Joyce and Lenin's manuscripts are swapped, art and politics being muddled in the process.[42] The fact that the manuscript-baby switch becomes a manuscript-manuscript switch symbolizes *Travesties*' intensified preoccupation with writing, and particularly the writing of history, as fictional. Written words have value, but that value does not lie in verity.

However, Stoppard is not intimidated by the unreliability of writing. Though the art war in his Zurich of 1917 is conducted primarily through words, it is presented as performance. Whether Lenin's speeches, Tzara's poetry readings, Joyce's production of *The Importance of Being Earnest* or Stoppard's own *Travesties*, performance is inextricably linked to the artist—and the politician's—attempts to communicate to their audiences. The historical Lenin was a rhetorician. His influence and power were built upon a talent for moving, persuading and inspiring large crowds. A string of successful dictators testify to this fact, and Stoppard, the dramatist, is only too keen to build upon it.

Performance also serves to further contain the proliferation of meaning discussed above as an aid to the defiance of radical relativism. As argued in reference to Hermione's resurrection scene in *The Winter's Tale* (Chapter 1), performance does away with many of the ambiguities a text may encourage. In performance, words cannot be regarded as detached, contextless scraps of paper; they are inevitably placed in a sequence of both words and actions. As Julia A. Walker argues:

> Unlike verbal signification, vocal signification can create, augment and/or reverse the presumed meaning of words by using pronunciation, tone coloration, and inflectional variation to speak to an emotional as well as conceptual register of "meaning." Similarly, pantomimic signification can create, augment, and/or reverse the presumed meaning of words by calling upon bodily comportment, gesture, and affect to speak to a spatio-temporal register of "meaning" as well . . . Meaning . . . *is* self-present. (Walker 2003: 160, 166)

By having his words spoken in performance—zany as that performance may be—Stoppard makes the meaning of his words self-present.

In order to understand what they see and hear, audiences must recognize the analogy between the theatrical stage and the stages of history, of Joyce's production of Wilde, of Carr's mind, and of their own cognitive makeup. Stoppard may not be interested in arousing a crowd to follow him personally in the political arena, but by demonstrating the inter(con)textual nature of art through drama, Stoppard forces his audience to confront the multiplicity of meaning, implicating his audiences in the process of meaning creation. Pearce reminds us that the viewer is integral to the process of mimesis. He goes so far as to claim that "We are all Narcissus. We cannot fully realize ourselves without the mirror. It is essential to us, and its essential nature encompasses our need to see ourselves in it" (Pearce 1145). As suggested above, few people in the audience are likely to see themselves in any of the play's characters, except perhaps in Carr as Everyman. But by seeing these characters reflected in the mirror of mimesis we are invited to assess our standpoint on the matters they discuss and to consider both their greatness and their folly through Stoppard's parody.

Heidegger already argued that which neurologists can now prove (Damasio 1999): we cannot relate to an object without engaging our thought; we automatically apprehend thoughtfully, and we cannot but be affected. Our relation to the world is always complex, multiple, temporal. Thus, whether or not we identify with Stoppard's characters, we cannot remain indifferent to them. This position has more recently been developed by Andy Clark, who corroborates Heidegger when he maintains that human perception does not map external reality so much as seek direction for active intervention: we see in "action-oriented representations" (Clark 1998: 276).[43] Further still, Heidegger's notion of "equipment" can be related to Clark's "wideware," a function that includes environmental elements that are not realized in either the brain or the central nervous system, but extend the cognitive system. These include different tactics we use to off-load information (such as making a list) so that "words, texts, symbols and diagrams often figure deeply in the problem-solving routine developed by the biological brains nurtured in language-rich environmental settings" (Clark 1998: 271). The dichotomy of subject/object is replaced by Heidegger's "Being-in-the-world" (1927: 207), a concept remarkably similar to Clark's "the-agent-in-the-world" (1998: 271). The subjective interpreter is always already in the world, and the world of objects exists as a web of structural relationships. In other words, of inter(con)textual activity.

This complements the claims made by cognitive linguist George Lakoff and philosopher Mark Johnson in their seminal work *Metaphors We Live By*. They argue that our everyday experience, as physical bodies, grounds our conceptual frameworks, including the very concept of framework. We conceive of metaphors such as "looking up" to someone or exercising "higher" faculties because we stand upright and our heads are, vertically, at the top, in a higher position; when we are depressed, physically or emotionally, we tend to bow down. There are "systematic correlates between our emotions (like happiness) and our sensory-motor experiences (like erect posture), these form the basis of metaphoric orientational concepts" (Lakoff and Johnson 1980: 58).

Our bodies shape metaphorical structures, but these, in turn, shape our (often unconscious) experience, which is mediated through cultural presuppositions. We interpret our sensations with the aid of a value-system that is largely culture-specific. A detailed example Lakoff and Johnson study, which is particularly relevant to *Travesties*, is our conception of "argument" as a kind of "war" (Lakoff and Johnson 1980: 4). They point out that we do not just talk about arguments in terms of war but "we see the person we are arguing with as an opponent. We attack his positions and we defend our own" (1980: 4). In other words, argument *is* war, a war of words. Both activities are structured by the same metaphoric conception. Nonetheless, metaphorical structuring is always partial. If the overlap were total, "one concept would actually be another, not merely be understood in terms of it" (1980: 13). Accordingly, argument differs from many wars not only in the means with which it is fought but because it cannot be perpetuated by an aggressor at the expense of a victim. Argument, ironically perhaps, relies upon the cooperation principle (Grice 1975) that binds both interlocutors in an agreement to stay and argue instead of leaving the room (or shooting the opponent, which would merge the different kinds of war-argumentation into one). Nonetheless, argument is not a purely cerebral activity. Heated arguments may elicit surprise, anger, stress, fear, or exhilaration—depending on the context—but they necessarily result in bodily affects: pulse racing and increased body-heat. Emotions, I repeat, are embodied.

By extension, Stoppard's play could never remain in the realm of language games without affecting his audiences' bodies. Audiences become interested in the different characters' arguments, are eager for one or other of the characters to triumph, and are finally satisfied when Joyce pulls off his successful coup, and when the couples promise to marry at the end. Feeling interested, eager and satisfied are all emotional responses. Moreover, in *Travesties*, the argument-is-war category-conflation is further complicated by the implication that it is also a kind of circus-act. Joyce's tactics ultimately triumph partly because of their intellectual force but, also, because they have such aesthetic force: he is the better performer.

Stoppard's drama may be wordy and his characters difficult to identify with, but his attention to the power of performance does not fall short of *The Winter's Tale* or *Our Country's Good* (Chapters 1 and 3). When the character of Lenin announces that, "To lose one revolution is unfortunate. To lose two would look like carelessness!" (*Travesties* 58), Stoppard's stage-directions stipulate that he echo Lady Bracknell's famous lines dressed as Dr. Chasuble (and Nadya as Miss

Prism; *Travesities* 53), while at the same time standing in a charismatic pose that reproduces the "justly famous image" of his public address to the Russian people in May 1920. In The Nottingham Playhouse's production of the play (2003),[44] the actor pronounced these words while standing on a table, (serving, presumably, as a substitute for the pedestals that would later support his statue in similar poses all over the Soviet Union), a bright red handbag dangling from his raised arm.[45] The quintessential symbol of Wilde's play is transformed into a citation of cabaret or even drag. This multi-layered visual statement serves not only to parody Lenin through a witty intertextual game, nor merely to echo much early twentieth-century art, but exemplifies the means by which *Travesties* draws upon the potential of performance. Language is understood to be inextricably linked to embodied experience—to the audiences' responses to performance.

Indeed, the OED affords the word "travesty" two main definitions: 1) a farcical or grotesque imitation; mockery; parody, and 2) the act of disguising (by dressing up); masking; cross-dressing. *Travesties* travesties history by re-presenting or re-dressing it, but it also makes significant use of outward appearances, costume, and disguise to illustrate their role in the creation of realities. Clothes, and especially trousers, are of great and recurring importance in Carr's dealings with the world (the military uniform of the British soldiers in France or Algernon's outfits), but they are also a means for Lenin to get back to Russia (disguises, wigs, and false IDs), Tzara to make art (the hat and coat pockets from which he produces his scraps of paper), and for Joyce to express his indifference to convention (the chronically mismatched suits). The fashioning of self, politics, and art are revealed to be greatly determined by outward show. Both the creation of identity, and its recognition by others, appear to be as much visual as conceptual. As John William Cooke notes, art and life are equally theatrical, equally designed for an external spectator: "the creation of self is a performance" (Cooke 1981: 536). By coming to see this performance, the audience in the theater is invited to partake in the process of meaning-creation, challenging the audience to exercise their creativity and realize their creative potential as artists.

VII. Conclusion

John Wood, the British actor who played the character of Henry Carr in the 1974 London production of *Travesties*, and whom Stoppard had in mind when writing the part, has explained that "in Tom's play the word is all. The word is beating back against the silence,

beating back the darkness. Thought is all we've got, says Tom, otherwise the dark, the jungle will close in on us" (Wood 1975; Delaney
1994).[46] This statement reveals that *Travesties* is specifically directed
at a Postmodern audience concerned with combating cynicism, pessimism, and unqualified skepticism.[47] It is important to note that,
though (literary) interpretation can escape the relativistic equation
by precluding the application of truth-falsity values altogether, lend-
ing itself to values such as admissible, apt, effective, or interesting
rather than true, that, nonetheless, even in art not all interpretations
are equally plausible or helpful. *Travesties* manages to express a wide
range of different approaches to art and its truth(s) but also shows
that, despite the fact that incongruent interpretations can share some
validity, not all are as convincing or as productive. Paradoxically,
though seeming to dramatize immoral, egocentric, and often-cynical
behavior—*Travesties* negates these traits. Stoppard claims that

> I want to write plays that are just funny enough to do their jobs but
> not *too* funny to obscure them. My line at the moment would be to
> try to reduce weighty preoccupations about the way the world is going
> to an extended exchange of epigrams with a good first-act curtain.
> (Stoppard to Bradshaw; Delaney 95–96)

Through an exploration of Stoppard's attitude to (avant-garde) performance it becomes apparent that his suggested cure for unqualified
skepticism is very similar to Shakespeare's: it lies in supplementing
philosophical knowledge with myriad other knowledge forms, and
in assuming responsibility for what Hosek and Freeman term one's
"actions into the world" (2001: 515). Stoppard celebrates active
engagement in and with the world. He rejects the idea of the artist
as detached onlooker; he pulls up his sleeves and plunges his hands
into the cauldron of life. By representing his world Stoppard claims
possession of it. He acknowledges that there is no one correct version
of reality, but he nonetheless claims dominion of *his* reality. As Claire
Colebrook suggests

> The idea that our world is always a represented world renders us both
> responsible for that world, at the same time as we recognize our sepa-
> ration or non-coincidence with the world. [. . .] If we acknowledge an
> essential separation of representation, then we also have to allow the
> question of who represents or what is demanding representation. [. . .]
> Acknowledging this minimal form of ownness or location of knowl-
> edge therefore entails that we cannot think of the world as writing

itself, giving itself or offering itself in a dispersed, anonymous or continuous representation. (Colebrook 60–63)[48]

The preoccupation with intellectual and artistic verbosity in *Travesties* is supplemented by its (necessarily spatio-temporal, visual, auditory) production on stage, which activates (and deliberately disorients) the audience's sense-perception. The physical presence of the actors on stage co-opts the audience's motor equivalence, and the skilful use of voice—inflection, volume, and song (all specified by the stage directions)—combine to create effects that far surpass the scope of language alone.

Travesties provides an alternative aesthetic to that of many Postmodernists, holding at its core a celebration of possibility, by demonstrating a worldview I have termed "cognitive inter(con)textuality." Ultimately, the various threads of Stoppard's artistic experimentalism express a vision of life-as-art, not in the sense of a detached wish-fulfilment but as a self empowering, liberating, infinitely rich, and positive assertion of the joy of existence. This affirmation is not a mere celebration of life in the face of fear and debilitating skepticism. Stoppard's play presents humans not as isolated individuals, doomed to live in lonely solipsism, nor as separate entities forever reaching for meaning just beyond our grasp. Instead, *Travesties* demonstrates that meaning is something we are at liberty to *create*. But this creation is necessarily a collaborative effort—a product of the interactive dynamics between bodies and words, texts and contexts, individuals and their environments, including other people. According to Stoppard, the construction and communication of meaning are the ultimate goals of the artist and may lead to no less than immortality.

Chapter 3

From Empathy to Sympathy: Staging Change and Conciliation in Timberlake Wertenbaker's *Our Country's Good*

All the members of human society stand in need of each others assistance, and are likewise exposed to mutual injuries. Where the necessary assistance is reciprocally afforded from love, from gratitude, from friendship, and esteem, the society flourishes and is happy. All the different members of it are bound together by the agreeable bands of love and affection, and are, as it were, drawn to one common center of mutual good offices.
(Smith 1759 Part II II.iii.1)[1]

Justice and humanness have never gone hand in hand. The law is not a sentimental comedy.
(Captain Watkin Tench, *Country* 3)

In 1788, Britain established a penal colony in New South Wales. By 1868, one hundred and sixty thousand convicts had been exiled to Australia. According to historical records, a few months after the first transportation arrived in the colony, a group of convicts was permitted to put on a play for the entertainment of the Marine officers in celebration of King George III's birthday. The play they performed was George Farquhar's *The Recruiting Officer*, a popular Restoration comedy with which the officers were almost certainly familiar. Captain Watkin Tench recorded in his journal:

> That every opportunity of escape from the dreariness and dejection of our situation should be eagerly embraced, will not be wondered at. The exhilarating effect of a splendid theater is well known: and I am not ashamed to confess that the proper distribution of three or four yards of stained paper, and a dozen farthing candles stuck around the mud walls of a convict hut, failed not to diffuse general complacency

on the countenance of sixty persons, of various descriptions, who were assembled to applaud the representation. (Tench 1793: 26/152)

It is surprising, however, that Captain Tench and his fellow officers do not seem to have deemed it remarkable that the performers of this "splendid theater" were convicts, recently exiled halfway across the earth to a labor camp. There remains, in fact, very scant documentation regarding the initiators and participants of this convict performance. In 1987, novelist Thomas Keneally felt inspired to write a novel, *The Playmaker*, in which he imagines how the performance may have come about. In the following year, 1988, The Royal Court Theater in London commissioned playwright Timberlake Wertenbaker to write a stage version of *The Playmaker*.[2]

Both Keneally and Wertenbaker imagine that, despite failing to mention it in their journals, the officers must have held some sort of discussion before the convict-production was sanctioned. In both *The Playmaker* and *Our Country's Good*, heated debates, confrontations, and violent interruptions precede the public performance of Farquhar's play, while the cooperation, empathy and self-articulation that emerge during rehearsals have astounding effects upon convicts and officers alike. Both texts present the convict-production as a transforming and redemptive experience. In other respects, however, novel and play differ markedly. Wertenbaker has largely overthrown Keneally's novel, using the story outline and characters he created only to the extent that they suit her own agenda. Thus, Wertenbaker leads her audience to reach very different conclusions from those reached by the novelist.

In this chapter I explore the means by which Wertenbaker dramatizes the possibility of defying radical skepticism, isolation, and despair and of encouraging trust in embodied receptiveness. Through interlacing Enlightenment and Sentimentalist theories into her play, Wertenbaker explores the role of sensibility, sentiments and emotional contagion in performance, suggesting that it may reconstruct damaged spirits and transform a heterogeneous, even hostile, group of individuals into a civic community in which respect, trust, and affection are possible. By testing the assumptions and processes Wertenbaker dramatizes in her play, I continue to pursue my underlying questions: can drama be trusted and, thus, (re)create trust? And, if so, how?

I. The Question of Liz: Learning to Articulate Sentiment

Having been "spewed" from their country for that "country's good," the convicts are presented in the opening scene of the play as having been reduced to near-animals, both by the harshness of their lives and by the brutalizing experiences of penal bondage. Crammed like live-stock into their transportation ship, they languish "alone, forgotten, nameless" (*Country* 1). The extent to which their humanity has been debased is made evident in their loss of language. The convicts have resorted to expressing their anger, fear, and despair through brutish grunts, beating, biting, barking, and loveless copulating. This back-drop makes the theatrical production of a refined and witty comedy about English gentry, written by a man of their (great)grandfather's generation, extremely challenging. Yet, within weeks of arriving at their destination, they find themselves 1) engaging with the polished language of *The Recruiting Officer*, 2) simulating a range of subtle emotions which they have not had the leisure to consider in their own lives for many years, if ever, 3) communicating effectively and 4) cooperating with one another in a group project. Soon the con-victs' common humanity and capacity for emotional complexity are emphasized over the bestial necessities of survival. The experience of participating in a theatrical production (re)introduces them to com-passion and trust.

In *Our Country's Good*, this process of regeneration and its pow-erful transformative effects do not come as a surprise to the liberal governor of the colony, Arthur Phillip. It is he who initiates the idea of putting on a play, precisely because he is convinced of the potential power of drama. Drawing inspiration from Socrates in Plato's dia-logue *The Meno*, Governor Phillip hopes that by teaching the con-victs refinement and language he will "*remind* the slave of what he knows, of his own intelligence...And by intelligence you may read goodness, talent, the innate qualities of human beings" (*Country* 57). In such remarks Philip also makes manifest his affiliations with the Sentimentalist trains of moral thought in his time, which viewed morality as grounded in an innate human disposition toward senti-ment; an inborn, natural benevolence which, if allowed to flourish, structures and anchors judgments.[3] Phillip's approach coheres with Adam Smith's assertion that

> The man who esteems himself as he ought, and no more than he ought, seldom fails to obtain from other people all the esteem that he himself thinks due. He desires no more than is due to him, and he rests upon it with complete satisfaction. (1759 Part VI I.iii.50)[4]

Thus, by improving the self-esteem of the convicts through empha-sizing their better qualities, the convicts will project a more positive image of themselves to others and, consequently, command the esteem of others.

Though the period known as the Enlightenment is usually discussed in terms of rational, scientific thinking and legal contractual philosophies (discussed below), these were accompanied by a fundamental interest in affective possibilities. Sentimentalism later became a pejorative term, often used to denoted excessive or foolish (and usually female) emotionality, but it began as an influential moral philosophy. Sentimentalism established new cultural norms and patterns of conduct, legitimizing emotions in both private and civic life and performing a general cultural (re)education by calling attention to, and demanding consideration of, emotions.

William Reddy explains that prior to 1700, "the role that emotions played in politics was as secondary as it was muted in relations between men and women" (Reddy 2000: 109). By 1789, the year of the French Revolution and, through historical coincidence, of the historical convict-production in New South Wales, a profound change had taken place in European attitudes. It had become widely accepted that "sincere emotions were of great political importance" (111). After the fall of Robespierre in 1794, and in response to the direction the revolution eventually took, emotions in politics were soon, once again, suspected.[5] But in the latter part of the eighteenth century, in the period that culminates just at the historical moment at which *Our Country's Good* is set, national obedience and loyalty were sought not merely through threatening fear-tactics but through inspiring a sense of shared interests, mutuality, and national identity. Wertenbaker's Governor Phillip's vision of society articulates a synthesis of Enlightenment principles matched with Sentimentalist moral standards. He envisages a rule of sensitivity, compassion, and education.

Because initially Wertenbaker's Governor Phillip describes convict Liz Morden as "lower than a slave, full of loathing, foul mouthed, desperate," it is clear that she is to be *the* test-case for his experiment, "to be made an example of" (*Country* 58). And indeed, during the course of the play, Liz moves from a passive acceptance of misery—"Luck? Don't know the word. Shifts its bob when I comes near" (*Country* 53)—to defiant hope. Her new sense of worth and legitimacy is expressed in her use of language. At first, though wrongly accused of theft, she refuses to speak at her trial and save herself from hanging because, she says, "It doesn't matter what you say. If they say you're a thief you're a thief" (*Country* 54). Through participating in the convict production Liz learns that what you say does matter.

In Act II.v Major Ross, the officer who most objects to the convict production, appears at a rehearsal and begins to humiliate each convict-actor in turn, trying to supersede their performance with his own exhibition of power. In desperation, convict Robert Sideway invites Liz to join him in performing the dramatic scene they have been rehearsing. By this stage in the play Liz has the self-possession and confidence to accept his invitation. Through acting out their parts, the convicts draw themselves out of passive obedience. Their text gives them the means with which to resist oppression, revealing a newfound solidarity among the actors. Dramatic production has forged bonds of friendship and trust where previously aggression, competition, suspicion, and isolation predominated. Hobbes' vision of a "state of nature" has undergone not merely a process of civilization, but one characterized by Sentimentalist convictions. Performance has also become a form of bold self-empowerment whereby Liz proves to herself that she can stand up to injustice.

How could such radical transformation have been effected? Let us first consider the specifically linguistic skills that the theatrical experience develops. Stanley Cavell argues that there are two stages to comprehension: knowing and acknowledging, for the former can occur without prompting the latter. As mentioned in Chapter 1, he argues that full acknowledgement entails "wording, the willingness to subject oneself to words, to make oneself intelligible" (Cavell 1987: 4). This view is enhanced by Andy Clark's assertion that language is "a mode of cognition-enhancing self-stimulation" (Clark 2006: 370); a "key cognitive tool enabling us to objectify, reflect upon, and hence knowingly engage with, our own thoughts, trains of reasoning, and personal cognitive characters" (372). Kay Young and Jeffery Saver concur, stretching the concept of language to encompass a larger consciousness of narrative form and progression. They maintain that "what predominates or fundamentally constitutes our consciousness is the understanding of self and world in story" (Young and Saver 2001: 73). Indeed, Roger Schank claims that "intelligence is bound up with our ability to tell the right story at the right time" (Schank 1990: 21).

Accordingly, it may be argued that by introducing Liz to language, and thus to the possibility of her own production of narrative, which also both elicits and articulates emotions, Governor Phillip is not simply attempting to impose culture upon her from above but to generate within her an internal process of self-articulation and identification, of self-construction. For a woman such as Liz it is a revelation to discover that she may influence, even rewrite, the script of her life.

Moreover, scientists seem to have been able to determine a link between the mirror-neuron system (MNS) and brain-regions involved in linguistic processing (Rizzolatti and Arbib 1998; Arbib 2005). Experiments show an overlap in activations of action-recognition and language-production areas of the brain (Molnar-Szakacs 2006: 933). Research indicates that the more one is exposed to demonstrations of complex actions and the more practice one gets in performing these actions oneself, the more one increases one's range of cognitive complexities. These complexities are registered in the very biological structures of the brain in both action-perception and language production areas concurrently (partly since these two seem to share the very same cognitive resources and neural substrata, Borca's area; Molnar-Szakacs 2006: 925).

In Act I, chained and humiliated, Liz speaks the language of the mistreated poor. And yet, by the time of her retrial, Liz is able to argue, defend, and even acquit herself. When she finally speaks to the Governor, her eloquence vindicates the hopes he held out for drama: "Your Excellency, I will endeavor to speak Mr. Farquhar's lines with the elegance and clarity their own worth commands" *(Country* 83). This remark is proof of conciliation. In contrast to the kind of treatment to which she has become accustomed, the governor shows Liz respect and sympathy and she rises to the occasion with gratitude. Most importantly, this scene presents a situation in which a convict's new language skills enable her to be *believed*. Language both provides the tools with which Liz explains herself and enables her to inspire genuine trust in her fellow humans. Moreover, the urgency of this sentiment echoes Smith's description of a universal human trait that may itself have produced the motivation for language:

> The desire of being believed, the desire of persuading, of leading and directing other people, seems to be one of the strongest of all our natural desires. It is, perhaps, the instinct upon which is founded the faculty of speech, the characteristical faculty of human nature. (1759: Part VII iv.25)

Liz's new skills have also, however, been interpreted very differently. Stephen Weeks does not contest that, at first, the convicts' distinct "lag-language" deepens the chasm between them and the society from which they have been expelled.[6] But he also argues that Liz can in fact speak the King's English from the start. He believes that she refuses to do so, rejecting her oppressors by rejecting their language. Such an interpretation implies that by participating in the convict production Liz does not acquire new language-tools with which to shape her own identity but, rather, acquires an understanding of the language-games of power manipulation. Weeks suggests that her final remark about speaking Farquhar's lines with elegance is spoken with knowing irony as expression of the triumph of "a convict underdog confronting the smug classist and sexist assumptions of the military tribunal" and "tends to read in performance as witty and self-possessed, even arrogant" (Weeks 2000: 148).

My experience of this scene in performance was very different and, moreover, this interpretation seems unlikely in light of the testimonies of the original colony officers. The historical Captain Watkin Tench mused in his journal that:

> A leading distinction, which marked the convicts on their outset in the colony, was an use of what is called the flash, or kiddy language. In some of our early courts of justice, *an interpreter was frequently necessary to translate the disposition of the witness, and the defense of the prisoner.* This language has many dialects. The sly dexterity of the pickpocket; the brutal ferocity of the footpad; the more elevated career of the highwayman; and the deadly purpose of the midnight ruffian, is each strictly appropriate in the terms which distinguish and characterize it. I have ever been of the opinion, that an abolition of this unnatural jargon would open the path to *reformation.* And my observations on these people have constantly instructed me, that indulgence in this infatuating cant, is more deeply associated with depravity, and continuance in vice, than is generally supposed. I recollect hardly one instance of a return to honest pursuits, and habits of industry, where this miserable perversion of our noblest and peculiar faculty was not previously conquered. (1793: 208, my italics)

In Act I, chained, beaten, and humiliated, Liz speaks the only language with which she is familiar. Her language at this time cannot be intended to express a conscious choice motivated by political ideology since she lacks both the sophistication and the strength of will required for such defiance. Unlike Hermione's silence in Act V of *The Winter's Tale*, Liz's silence only marks her weariness and resignation to injustice. And yet, by the end of her retrial, after she has undergone—quite literally—a dramatic metamorphosis, Liz is not only grateful and relieved that the court has acquitted her but has internalized her right to fair hearing (*Country* 83). This is the fundamental reversal. Her response to the governor is not petty vindictiveness but genuine gratitude. This is so very optimistic a claim, and so close a dramatization of eighteenth-century Sentimentalist views, that some viewers may find it incredible, but it is true to the claims Wertenbaker makes for drama in her play.[7]

Demonstrations of emotional stress, such as sighing, fainting, and crying, have always been suspected of questionable sincerity, and expressions of overpowering emotions (whether in the melodramas of the time or today) are often considered, at best, embarrassing. But serious consideration of the role of emotions in private and public life must necessarily also entail displays of emotion. The fine line between affection and affectation must always be minded, but it is a mark of contemporary cynicism that Liz is suspected of the latter, when Wertenbaker tries so unashamedly to present the former. Contemporary critics, particularly at the time the play was first performed, at the high point of Margaret Thatcher's role as Prime Minister,[8] and before the collapse of the Communist block, may be excused for worrying that even if Liz is genuinely grateful, this gratitude is a sign of her ongoing oppression disguised as benevolence. This is not, however, how Wertenbaker presents it. Whether or not the individual viewer is convinced by Philosophical Sentimentalism, its premises are those Governor Phillip endorses and those which Wertenbaker herself eagerly dramatizes.[9]

In Act I.vi Governor Phillip reminds his officers that attending a play was considered by the Greeks to be a "kind of work in that it required attention, judgment, patience, all social virtues" (*Country* 22). Captain Tench retorts:

> *Tench*: And the Greeks were conquered by the more practical Romans, Arthur.
> *Collins*: Indeed the Romans built their bridges, but they also spent many centuries wishing they were Greeks. And they, after all, were conquered by barbarians, or their own corrupt and small spirits.
> *Tench*: Are you saying Rome would not have fallen if the theater had been better?
> *Ralph*: (*very loud*) Why Not? . . .

It is reasonable to assume that Wertenbaker intends a touch of irony here, but the convictions she places in the mouths of Ralph Clark and Governor Phillip are the convictions that triumph in her play.

Nonetheless, considering her importance as the focal test-case of the play, it may come as a surprise to learn that the character of Liz is entirely invented by Wertenbaker. Liz is the only character who has no basis in history, nor is she borrowed from Keneally's novel.[10] In the novel, the part of Malinda in *The Recruiting Officer* is played by

Nancy Turner. Unlike the graceless Liz, Nancy possesses "the dark, erotic malice of her character Malinda" (Keneally 1987: 42). She is dubbed "Turner the Perjurer" for having lied in court to save her lover, Marine private Dukes. He is hanged with five others nonetheless, but she is acquitted at her own trial when the main witness against her is disqualified. At this trial she remains silent, but her motives are entirely different from those attributed to Liz in the play. Indeed, at the end of the novel we discover that Nancy did not commit perjury at her lover's trial but, rather, spoke the truth knowing that she would be disbelieved. Thus, paradoxically, through cunning manipulation of the court, she rids herself of an undesired ex-lover, even though he is, as testified, innocent. As Keneally's Ralph sees it, Nancy's behavior exemplifies "the mystery of criminal purpose" (342). This conclusion is far from the one to which Wertenbaker leads us. In itself, therefore, Liz's story cannot be considered "proof" that language and drama may reform damaged souls, and Wertenbaker's choice of the name Liz, likely intended to remind the audience of Eliza Doolittle in Shaw's *Pygmalion* (1913), only enhances the fictionality of her tale.

What then may we make of Wertenbaker's analogy between linguistic dexterity and personal empowerment? Cavell believes the best means of accessing the essences of the world is through language and "a sense of the intimacy of words with the world, or of intimacy lost." Similarly, through his rule of compassion and sensibility, Wertenbaker's Governor Phillip leads convicts and officers alike to develop a love of language that enables accuracy, intimacy, and rigor. Wording the world is shown to be of crucial importance. Moreover, cognitive psychologists now maintain that, though we are naturally disposed to feel, many specific emotions are learned. Stephen Turner has shown that some complex emotions, such as angst or belief, are *learned* together with the words that describe them in a particular culture (Turner 2000: 114). If effusions of sympathy are cultivated, then Phillip is not merely acknowledging responses that are already there yet denied but, rather, allowing them to develop and intensify, where previously they may have been stifled or even absent. Thus, as I have been suggesting in this book, expressions of feeling in literature, and particularly in drama, play an important role in the emotional education of readers, participants, and viewers.

In *Our Country's Good*, Major Ross ardently opposes Governor Philip, but he does so in surprisingly musical and comically alliterative language. Ross expects the "frippery frittering play" (*Country* 19), combined with the "threatening theory" encouraged by theater (*Country* 25), to bring "calamity on this colony" (*Country* 51). On the other hand his sidekick, Captain Jemmy Campbell, is less articulate than most convicts and expresses his agreement with Ross through comments such as "Eh, kev, weh, discipline's bad" (*Country* 17). Wertenbaker's Ross remains steadfastly strict and brutal throughout. But Campbell—perhaps because of his deficient powers of articulation—reveals a susceptibility to the effects of the convicts' play. At the end of Act I, when Ross comes to the first rehearsal to inform Ralph that "five men have run away and it's all because of your damned play" (*Country* 51), he delivers his message and then immediately leaves, a sign of his understanding of the dramatic importance of exiting while the audience is awestruck. Campbell lingers on, looking at the play-text: "Ouusstta. *The Recruiting Officer*. Good title. Arara. But a play, tss, a play" (*Country* 52). In Act II, when Ross and Campbell deliver the newly recaptured Caesar and Morden to their rehearsal bound in chains, Campbell is swept up by the rehearsal, showing interest in Farquhar's lines: "Mmhem, good, that. Sighs, vows, promises, hehem, mmm. Anxieties" (*Country* 65). Ross puts an immediate stop to this by commanding him to start Arscott's flogging. But when in II.x Ross complains of the corrupting effects of the play, which shows officers lying and cheating, Campbell cannot resist admitting that "Good scene that, very funny, hah, scchhh," and eagerly quotes from the text of the play, until he is once again silenced by Ross (*Country* 81). Were he allowed to participate in the convict-production, it is quite possible that Campbell would undergo similar transformations to those the convict-actors undergo.

One of literature's greatest epistemic contributions resides in its aesthetic merits. Adam Smith, for instance, argued that "the poets and romance writers, who best paint the refinements and delicacies of love and friendship, and of all other private and domestic affections" are "much better instructors than Zeno, Chrysippus, or Epictetus" (1759 Part III iii.14). But literary articulation, by affording new forms of language construction and thought extension, goes beyond argumentation and reaches realms of expression that may reconfigure past beliefs, or generate new ones. As Tzachi Zamir asserts, "We do not merely arrive at more thoughts of the same kind that we had before. Rather, aesthetic articulation enables gaining a hold on life's essentials, maintaining connections with evasive moments that escape us as they create what is most important" (Zamir 2007: 29). Fiction suggests new patterns through which to comprehend possibilities and engage with them.

And yet, the language, the plot, and the characters of *The Recruiting Officer* are not so very profound or unique that they, in themselves, explain the effect of the play upon the convicts dramatized in *Our Country's Good*. This fact lends credence to the hypothesis that their production-experience must have tapped into a subtler and more direct form of learning. I suggest that this form of learning is natural, instinctive, and body-based: an appeal to the senses that accesses pre-conscious embodied receptiveness.

II. Teaching the Body: (Theatrical) Simulation and Empathy

Jonathan Levy has rightly voiced concern that "what we currently call empathy means at least three things" (Levy 1997: 181).[11] I find his distinction between *Involuntary Emotional Identification*, *Sympathetic Projection*, and *Sympathetic Understanding* very productive, not least because it reminds us that not all three categories are co-present whenever the term empathy is evoked. As Jean Decety reminds us, though mirror neurons have been shown to affect motor systems and resonance, they have not yet been conclusively tied to the generation of emotions, and "it is not at present possible to conclude that [the mirror neuron system] is critically involved in emotion recognition" (Decety 2010: 2). Nonetheless, the discussion of empathetic potentialities in this book covers all three of Levy's categories and, furthermore, suggests that the core of the issue may lie in chronology. Just as reasoned analysis comes after the initial impact of emotion, so too sympathetic projection and understanding come after the initial impact of empathy. The involuntary, physical, mirror-resonance that defines empathy need not necessarily lead to sympathy; but sympathy is best achieved through eliciting empathy.

At the beginning of *Our Country's Good*, Officer Ralph Clark refuses to identify with a convict's subject position, asserting categorically that "I am not a convict: I don't sin" (*Country* 37). When Ketch tries to explain how he was mistakenly convicted and later coerced into accepting the job of colony hangman, he appeals to Ralph by asking, "what would you have done?" Ralph replies bluntly: "I wouldn't have been in that situation" (*Country* 37). The convicts are just as unpracticed in empathy or sympathy as the officers. When Liz at first rushes through her lines without impersonating Malinda, Ralph, having been appointed the director of the convict-production, suggests she imitates rich ladies she has seen in London. But Liz claims she never really observed the women, only their purses. When Ralph tries to conjure them in the context of the grand houses in which she had spied them, Liz can only evoke her sense of injustice: "it's not normal when others have nothing." When Ralph then says that she must try to imagine herself a rich lady, she begins to masticate. "What are you doing?" he asks in dismay. "If I was rich," she replies, "I'd eat myself sick" (*Country* 48).[12]

In order to bypass Liz's resistance to the character of Malinda, Ralph finally places a little piece of wood in her hand and pronounces it her fan. In response, Liz automatically adopts the standard accompanying ladylike posture. By performing an action—circumventing the conceptual and discursive registers of pretending to be a lady—Liz's body allows her to engage in a way her conscious mind cannot. Experience disrupts epistemological categories, successfully producing flexibility and change. Wertenbaker thus demonstrates how we may learn through the body and how drama facilitates and intensifies this process. Indeed, by the end of *Our Country's Good,* both convicts and officers are opened up to the existence and legitimacy of other subject positions.

Wertenbaker's dramatic heritage and personal intuition allow her, just as they allowed Shakespeare before her, to dramatize that which theorists regarded until recently with skepticism. Paul Ekman's research suggested in the early 1980s that certain basic facial expressions are universally recognized as expressing a set of specific human emotions. These include fear, happiness, surprise, sadness, anger, and disgust.[13] Regardless of ethnic or cultural backgrounds, these facial displays are instantaneously and universally comprehensible, providing a common starting point for intersubjective communication. Current science now informs us that interpretation then follows through attunement to the physical condition of others: through simulation and motor equivalence and the activation of memory-related CDZs, discussed in the introduction to this book. As mentioned in that discussion, simulation involves neither overt knowledge nor conscious inference but is achieved by *physical participation in observed action.* The extent to which Wertenbaker demonstrates these arguments is striking. The convict-actors undergo such profound changes through the dramatic production experience not merely because it develops their conscious, intellectual skills (articulation, argumentation, presentation) but because their bodies are in effect reprogrammed.

It is reasonable to assume that, with the new words they learn, Wertenbaker's convicts also learn new sentiments. But these sentiments are developed into a new approach to both self and com-munity through simulation. Turner asserts that "actual experiences, notably the empirical experiences gained in role-playing, imitation and simulation tested by experience, provide a great deal of the kind of psychological content that is needed to have the capacity to interact socially" as well as both foster and understand complex and subtle emotions (117). Through role-play we can accomplish some of what Spolsky describes as "fill[ing] in the gaps between kinds of knowl-edge" (Spolsky 2001a: 11).

While the convicts are speechless at first, Officer Ralph Clark is all words—reading the bible, writing his journal, writing to his wife.[14] For his spirit to be freed, he must be liberated *from words*.[15] By directing and taking part in *The Recruiting Officer* (as Captain Plume) Ralph is surprised to discover that, in return for his gift of words, the convict women teach him of embodied receptiveness. Dabby announces at their first meeting that she may not be able to read "those marks in the books" but she offers Ralph a barter deal: "Mary will read me the lines and I, Lieutenant, will read you your dreams" (*Country* 16). Later she tells Ralph: "I see things very clearly and I'm making you see clearly, Lieutenant" (*Country* 75). Gradually, Ralph learns to reweigh the significance of words by beginning to listen to—and value—the body, initiating a reverse-process that both mirrors and supplements the process the convicts undergo. This bi-directional process enables Ralph and Mary Brenham to fall in love, combining articulate sentiments with sensitive and sensual love.[16]

The scene of excitement in which Ralph and Mary meet as lov-ers on the beach and acknowledge their equal standing, stripped of the burdens of past officer-convict animosity, of their own past identities, of civilization, of false moralities, embodies the antithesis of the savage sex described aboard the convict-ships in Act I. But neither is this an example of the kind of stage-romance they enact in *The Recruiting Officer*. This scene confirms Spolsky's claims for the pastoral genre, detailed in Chapter 1. During the course of *Our Country's Good*, England's civilization, from which the convicts have been expelled, is exposed as ruthless, cruel, and at the same time frivolous and superficial. In contrast, the coast of Australia, where a merciless penal existence was to punish the convicts and force them to accept society's values, is transformed instead into an almost uto-pian "green-world" in which the convicts are not merely reformed but transformed. However, in a significant deviation from conven-tions, the heroes of this pastoral do not return to the old society but build a new one. They reject England's warped values, erase its prejudices and learn to see one another as human beings rather than social stereotypes.[17] The Governor wishes the convicts to "think in a free and responsible manner" (*Country* 21) so they can become true citizens of a new democratic republic. And, as the audience knows well, Australia indeed became just that.

In this scene, Wertenbaker echoes core Sentimentalist principles, such as the belief in connections between virtue and simplicity, sincerity and truth,[18] and echoes the increasingly democratic views expressed at that time. A century earlier, John Locke had asserted that God created all men free and equal. In his *Two Treatises of Government*, he argues that since we are "born to all the same advantages of nature, and the use of the same faculties" we should also "be equal one amongst another without subordination or subjugation" (1689: ii.4: 101); this is "equality of men by nature" (1689: ii.5: 101). Human bodies are never identical, but we all have bodies and, whether we are conscious of it or not, share a basic understanding of one another's bodies. In turn, each character in *Our Country's Good* explores a different facet of the essential integration between body, emotion, and mind in the process of affecting change and acquiring satisfying knowledge. Wertenbaker argues thereby that a certain level of proficiency in both linguistic and physical modes of expression and reception are necessary for a harmonious existence. Both Liz Morden and Ralph Clark are thoroughly unbalanced individuals in Act I. By the end of *Our Country's Good* they have achieved a new level of personal peace.

Such claims are underscored by recent developments in clinical psychology. Psychologists now distinguish two categories of emotion: "basic emotions" and "moral emotions" (Olatunji 2007: 281).[19] "Basic emotions"—such as fear or disgust—entail distinct behavioral, cognitive, and physiological dimensions that are motor-sensory. They are registered in BOLD, that is, Blood-Oxygen-Level-Dependency signals. These can be activated without particular neurons firing and, thus, without registering in our consciousness. "Moral emotions," on the other hand, are distinguished by "their linkage to the interest or welfare of society as a whole or of persons other than the judge or agent" (Moll et al. 2005: 68). "Moral emotions" do invade our consciousness and are influenced by cultural assumptions and personal preferences of a moral kind. In other words, moral emotions assume different properties and affect different bodily regions from the strictly-sensory basic emotions, but they are, nonetheless, just as embodied. Thus, as any good advertiser or propagandist knows, moral emotions may be unconsciously acquired and subliminally affected through the manipulation of basic, embodied response mechanisms.

Elsewhere I have written about the dangerous ends which this propensity may serve but, in the present context, this dynamic is used to instigate positive change.[20] The metamorphosis experienced by the convict-actors is brought about by a combination of factors including, as noted above, language skills. But their receptiveness to the *moral values* the Governor wishes to teach is generated by accessing their pre-conscious, bodily receptors. And these, in turn, are accessed through participation in the convict-production.

Dramatic production has indeed been shown to modify behavioural patterns. Performance theorist Richard Schechner has argued for some years that, when reproducing facial expressions we often also reproduce the correlating emotions. His theories aim to explains how the rigorous facial exercises undertaken by young Indian boys as part of their training for kathakali dance theater, though wholly artificial "mechanical" maneuvers, can be conducive to very profound learning (Schechner 1988: 264).[21] Liz's experience with the prop fan may be fictional, but it matches Schechner's claim that performance regularly affects neurological systems, effecting deep emotional learning that bypasses intellectual engagement.

Schechner's claims for the theater have since been tested in the laboratory. Damasio asserts that emotions can create effects, stored in the body, which do not have an associated image or memory (which requires narration), generating a preference for particular action or behavior patterns that are commensurate with the emotional value of the original emotional encounters (Damasio 1999: 46). Emotional response generates a different type of knowledge and a different type of memory. In addition, "we do not need to be conscious of the inducer of an emotion and often are not, and we cannot control emotions willfully" (47). That is, we cannot will them into being, or will them away. Nonetheless, stipulates Damasio, "if the psychological and physiological context is right, an emotion will ensue" (48). This implies that if the specific expression related to one of the six basic emotions is deliberately assumed, the correlating emotion should also arise.

Schechner also refers to Michael D. Gershon's *The Second Brain* (1998), according to which there is a brain in the belly:

The gut's brain, known as the enteric nervous system [ENS], is located in sheaths of tissue lining the esophagus, stomach, small intestine, and colon. Considered a single entity, it is a network of neurons, neurotransmitters, and proteins that zap messages between neurons, support cells like those found in the brain proper and a complex circuitry that enables it to act independently, learn, remember, and, as the saying goes, produce gut feelings. [...] Until relatively recently, people thought that the gut's muscles and sensory nerves were wired directly to the brain...they were surprised to find that the gut contains 100 million neurons—more than the spinal cord has. Yet the vagus nerve only sends a couple of thousand nerve fibers to the gut. (Schechner 2001:35–7)

The presence and location of the ENS confirms a basic principal of Asian medicine, meditation, and martial arts, "that the region in the gut between the navel and the pubic bone is the center/source of readiness, balance, and reception" (Schechner 2001: 38). Hiadt reinforces the claim that the bowls reflect "the operation of a second brain" and explains that this brain is possessed of "a high degree of autonomy" from the head-brain and even continues to function well even if the vagus nerve, which connects the two brains together, is severed. In line with Schechner's claims, Haidt hypothesizes that:

The independence of the gut brain, combined with the autonomic nature of changes in the genitals, probably contributed to ancient Indian theories in which the abdomen contains the three lower chakras—energy centers corresponding to the colon/anus, sexual organs, and gut. The gut chakra is even said to be the source of gut feelings and intuitions, that is, ideas that appear to come form somewhere outside one's own mind. (Haidt 2006: 6–7)

These claims correspond further with the cognitive theories outlined in the introduction to this book, which suggest that the brain works in conjunction with other neural networks and peripheral nervous system pathways stretching all over the body. The production, recognition and recollection of emotions require cooperation between multiple cerebral systems that extend into various parts of the body proper. (Note, once again, that the brain is itself a part of the body). As Damasio explains, there is no single emotional brain-site but rather "discrete systems related to separate emotional patterns" (62).[22]

Even more crucial to the present argument is the understanding that "imitation is a highly complex cognitive process, involving vision, perception, representation, memory and motor control [...] Learning by imitation, like any cognitive process, must be considered an intrinsically embodied process" (Borenstein and Ruppina 2005: 229–230). There appears to be "a universal and fundamental link between the ability to replicate the actions of others (imitation) and the capacity to represent and match others' actions (mirroring)"

(239–40). Furthermore, experiments show that observation is not sufficient to learn complex tasks.[23] Education, as Zuckow-Goldring and Arbib note, involves drawing attention to the most relevant factors, by directing "educated attention" to specific evidence; "the novice can build up new skills by assisted, complex, goal-directed imitation, rather than an incredibly protracted process of trial and error" (Zuckow-Goldring and Arbib 2007: 2184–85). This, I submit, is precisely the kind of work literature, and drama in particular, advances. Attention-directing interactions, gestures, verbal displays, and physical simulation (performance and practice) speed up learning processes.

This process is made manifest in the re-education performed upon Leontes in *The Winter's Tale* by time, reflection, and Paulina's orchestration of Hermione's dramatic performance, and upon the convicts in *Our Country's Good* by their dramatic education. It is entirely possible that the convict-actors learn from Farquhar's characters, not by attempting to impersonate them convincingly for some performance but through their necessarily embodied interaction with these characters. The fact that they know perfectly well that they are not gentry makes little difference in this respect. The body learns its own lessons.

Wertenbaker's intuitions have also been put to the test: *Our Country's Good* has contributed to empirical verification of its own intuitive claims. In 1989, a group of prisoners serving life sentences put on *Our Country's Good* at Blundeston Prison in London.[24] Wertenbaker and most of the Royal Court cast attended the performance. Wertenbaker wrote afterward, "It seemed to me the play had come full circle, performed in that prison room with an intensity and accuracy playwrights dream of and I remember relishing the wit with which the prisoners portrayed the officers of the play."[25] Later that year, Wertenbaker received a letter from Joe White (prisoner no. N55463, D Wing), saying, "Drama and self-expression in general is a refuge and one of the only real weapons against the hopelessness of these places." He declares that theater has provided a "bridge" from institutionalized confinement to life, giving him "a certain degree of confidence and genuine optimism;" both "maintaining and consolidating a more personal sense of worth and purpose." The testimonies of Joe and other Blundeston lifers indicate that Wertenbaker's view of drama is no empty ideal.

The experience of participating in the production of *Our Country's Good* was no less metamorphosing than the one play itself dramatizes. Just like Wertenbaker's eighteenth-century convicts,

Blundeston's twentieth-century prisoners were trained to see themselves as legitimate people, rather than mere prisoners; to find their own voice and to articulate that voice in a way that enables them to be heard. It is known that some of the convicts dramatized in *Our Country's Good* later became "Australia's first actors, theater managers and writers" (Inverso 1993: 422). In turn, some of the lifers who took part in *Our Country's Good* at Blundeston prison also continued thereafter to read, write, and put on plays. In fact, after his release, Joe White worked as assistant director for the 1998 production of *Our Country's Good* at The Young Vic in London.

Interestingly, *Our Country's Good* is itself the product of a "Joint Stock" workshop conducted by playwright, director Max Stafford Clark, and actors, in which improvisation and discussion were germane to the shaping of the play. The company also both met with Keneally and travelled to Shrewsbury (the location of *The Recruiting Officer*). As part of their research they also attended another performance by prisoners at Wormwood scrubs (Stafford-Clark 24–29 cited in Carlson 1993: 275). The play is, thus, a product of both collaboration and compromise—a multi-vocal conglomerate of opinions—just like the production it dramatizes. Further yet, the original 1988 London production of *Our Country's Good* was a double-bill with *The Recruiting Officer*. The plays were performed on alternate nights, highlighting the play's intertextual influences. Thus Keneally and Farquhar were acknowledged as active participants in this extensive group project.

The evidence presented here suggests that, through role-play, language games, and performance techniques, drama's subtlety and indirectness can divert actors' attentions away from themselves and towards their roles, so that enmities, prejudices, and anxieties may be set aside for a while, while others are worked through. Actors thus, simultaneously, both forget and (re)discover themselves. At the same time, the activity of performing their roles teaches the performers' bodies' new lessons. We already know that "the body, through its motor abilities, its actual movements, and its posture, informs and shapes cognition" (Gallagher 2005: 8). As I have been claiming throughout this book, drama both induces emotion and brings to the foreground awareness of emotion, its causes, and its consequences. This explains both how participating in the production of *The Recruiting Officer* could have had such a profound effect upon the convicts in *Our Country's Good* and how the performance of *Our Country's Good* could have affected contemporary British prisoners so deeply. The convicts free both their minds and their bodies from the restrictions of real and imagined chains in the process. In turn, when the audience views the actions played out before them, their brains and bodies also process, respond, and learn.

III. Staging Change: Performing Conciliation

Wertenbaker accentuates artifice in *Our Country's Good,* deliberately undermining the audiences' "suspension of disbelief." For instance, she specifies in the play's directions that there should be only ten actors for twenty-two characters. Thus, the actors often change costumes for their different parts on stage, women sometimes playing the parts of men. The tactic of constantly reminding the audience that those on stage are acting is hardly new. Neither is the doubling of parts technique. However, in *Our Country's Good,* the fact that downtrodden convicts are transformed into self-satisfied officers by an actor's swift alteration of costume, dramatizes the externality of the divisions between them. Because the same actor embodies such different characters, the audience is stuck by the fragility of role distinctions. Through a slight shift in circumstances or luck, each one of the officers could have been forced into crime and ended up a convict. Harry makes this explicit in Act I when he muses: "Sometimes I look at the convicts and I think, one of those could be you, Harry Brewer, if you hadn't joined the Navy when you did" (*Country* 7).

The audience is able to follow these role shifts because of their innnate mechanisms of simulation. As Julia A. Walker observes, audiences are made to recognize that "a single body can be comprehended through multiple discursive frames, a recognition that, significantly, comes to them through conceptual, affective, and experiential registers of 'knowledge'" (Walker 2003: 171).[26] The role-doubling technique further engages the audience's embodied receptiveness by constantly reminding us of the diversity of the actors' skills, equally able to convince us of both the characters they play. This, just as it does in the resurrection scene in *The Winter's Tale,* makes a consciously self-reflexive comment about the power of theatricality to advance human cognition.

As well as serving as a performance strategy, doubling of parts is also presented as a forced necessity in this play. Major Ross, who objects to the convict production, refuses to allow more that ten prisoners off work, especially not in order to replace Arscott, who tried to escape.[27] Some of the convicts must therefore play several parts in *The Recruiting Officer.* "It'll confuse the audience" worries Wisehammer. "Nonsense," replies Ralph, they will easily tell the parts apart "if they're paying attention." But "what if they aren't paying attention?" persists Wisehammer. "People who can't pay attention should not go to the theater" concludes Ralph (*Country* 73). Doubling, he argues, will challenge and train the audience's imagination. And as Dabby soon after asserts, "people with no imagination shouldn't go to the theater" (*Country* 75).[28]

The importance of the physicality of experience stressed further through constant reminders of the pain inflicted upon the convicts' bodies by brutal punishments, their constant pangs of hunger, and their longing for tenderness. This was made wonderfully visible in the stage design of both the Royal Court (1988) and Old Vic (1998) productions of the play in London, both sanctioned by the playwright. There were very few props—a few wooden boxes, a rope swing, a table, and basic costumes. Instead, the actors' bodies were the focal presence on the stage as well as the focal argument of the play. In turn, the audience's response to the play is conditioned by empathy, an engagement with the bodies of the characters and their performers.

Wertenbaker's awareness of theatrical effect is also expressed in her generic choice. The changes she makes to her characters create comedy where there was none. Keneally's novel is tremendously moving but not particularly funny. By making both Ralph and Campbell characters of far greater comic value than they are in the novel, by adding whole scenes, such as Liz's mastication scene, which afford comic relief and, most important, by choosing to end the play on a triumphant and optimistic note, Wertenbaker transforms her source material into comedy.[29] What does she hope to achieve by this?

In Sir Philip Sidney's *Defence of Poesie* (1595), it is asserted, "Tragedy maketh kings fear to be tyrants." Hamlet recounts this humanist theory:

> ...—Hum I have heard
> That guilty creatures sitting at a play,
> Have by the very cunning of the scene,
> Been struck so to the soul that presently
> They have proclaimed their malefactions. (II.ii.545–549)

Shakespeare's tyrant Claudius is indeed affected by Hamlet's play *The Mousetrap*, so much so that he leaves the room "marvelous distempered" (III.ii.275) and rushes to the chapel to pray. In this respect, the play is successful, since it convinces Hamlet of Claudius's guilt. However, crucially, Claudius does not abandon his tyranny. On the contrary, he abandons religion and plots to kill the playwright (Hamlet). Hamlet tests the humanist ideal and finds it a failure; the Machiavellian tyrant is resistant to the ethical claims of either religion or art. As Jeffrey Perl has pointed out, "Humanist dramaturgy does not succeed with a real audience" (Perl 1989: 9). Is, then, the humanist, and specifically Sentimentalist ideal, which Wertenbaker is so eager to promulgate, a question of genre? It appears that Wertenbaker thinks so.

Wertenbaker goes so far as to represent the stage as a substitute for the gallows. While contemporary Western audiences may by and large be relied upon to find public execution disturbing, in earlier centuries such events were not only well-attended but often considered a kind of comedy. In *Our Country's Good*, Captain Tench describes the "spectacle of hanging" as the convicts' "favorite form of entertainment" (*Country* 3). Governor Phillip suggests that perhaps the convicts have "never been offered anything else" as entertainment (*Country* 4). To make her point, Wertenbaker has Ketch Freeman, the colony's reluctant executioner, recall, while measuring Liz for hanging, "the terrible mess" at the execution of poor Tom Barrett, only seventeen: "It took twenty minutes and even then he wasn't dead. Remember how he danced and everyone laughed" (*Country* 67).[30] In the play, execution is forestalled by dramatic performance: participating in the convict-production enables Liz to save herself from hanging. And, through enacting his role as Justice Balance in *The Recruiting Officer*, Ketch Freeman is finally accepted by the community of players. Like Leontes in *The Winter's Tale*, Ketch allows the forgiveness of others to teach him self-forgiveness. In the last scene of *Our Country's Good*, Liz and Ketch stand side-by-side, ready to ascend the stage to perform a stage-comedy instead of the farcical tragedy of execution.

In the epigraph I chose for this chapter, Captain Watkin Tench declares, "Justice and humanness have never gone hand in hand. The law is not a sentimental comedy" (*Country* 3). However, in the play, we discover that the performance of a comedy may assist the profound redressing of injustices hitherto perpetuated by the law. The convict production does not turn the law into a joke; it overturns a conception of the law as a penal instrument, and creates a new vision of the law as one that serves to promote education, reform, democratic government, and public good. Such an act is, of course, grounded in the revolutionary political climate of the time. Thus, Wertenbaker's play may well be described as a sentimental comedy or, perhaps, to be more accurate, a Sentimentalist comedy.

IV. Two Contracts: Civic Order, Social Cohesion and Personal Freedom

In *Our Country's Good*, Wertenbaker draws parallels between the conduct required of the participants of a play and the conduct required of the citizens of a republic, revealing a political agenda which complements and extends her claims for drama. As opposed to the mass gathering described in the novel, and the ambitions expressed by Wertenbaker's Phillip for reforming the convict-community through providing them with cultured entertainment, historical records indicate that, in reality, the governor and officers of the garrison alone attended the convict performance in 1789. Moreover, it appears that the entire event was a convict initiative and an entirely convict-run project. Nowhere do historical documents mention Ralph or any other officer as director. Keneally may have chosen to have an officer-director in his novel in order to allow for a deeper and more interesting exploration of convict-officer relations but Wertenbaker goes a step further. In her play, Governor Arthur Phillip is the motivating force behind the convict-production and it is Phillip who insists on casting Liz as Malinda (*Country* 59). Keneally's colonial viceroy, referred to as H. E. (His Excellency), is concerned with "straight moral matters—...stealing deceiving and whoring; the secular virtues of reasonableness, obedience, and industry" (36). H. E. is repeatedly described as craving "social order" (49) and aspiring to a "rational kingdom" (112). Most of his subjects look to him for "sanity and hope" (104). But H. E. is not the experimental theater advocate that Phillip is in *Our Country's Good*.

In this respect, Keneally's viceroy is closer to historical records, as there exists no evidence that Arthur Phillip was in any way involved in the convict production, though he did attend the performance. In *The Playmaker*, Ralph is the main protagonist; Ralph's perspective and his experiences shaping the events recounted. Indeed Keneally's Ralph is also very different from the timid, effeminate, even ridiculous man Wertenbaker presents in her Act I. Keneally's Ralph is passionate: about his wife, about the play, about life. His pride in playmaking is evident from the very start. Moreover, the historical viceroy does not seem to have written a journal but there exists a book in The British Library, credited to him (though almost certainly not written by him), which states that on March 7, 1788, The Royal Commission was officially read out at a ceremony, declaring Phillip "Captain General and Governor in chief in and over the territory called New South Wales" (Phillip 1789: 64).[31] In his speech he informs the convicts that:

> by the lenity of [their country's] laws, they were now so placed that, by industry and good behavior they might in time regain the advantages and estimation is society of which they had deprived themselves. They not only had every encouragement to make that effort, but were removed almost entirely from every temptation to guilt. There was little in this infant community which one man could plunder from another, and any dishonest attempts in so small a society would almost infallibly be discovered. To persons detected in such crimes, he could not promise any mercy; nor indeed to any who under the circumstances, should presume to offend against the peace and good order of the settlement. (66)

However, he added, and this is of crucial importance: "those whose behavior should in any degree promise reformation, might always depend upon encouragement fully proportioned to their deserts" (67). And he concluded his address by declaring his "earnest desire to promote the happiness of all who were under his government, and to render the settlement in New South Wales advantageous and honorable to his country" (67).[32]

Echoes of Godwin, Bentham, and Smith cannot be overlooked here, such as Smith's firm belief that

> Concern for our own happiness recommends to us the virtue of prudence: concern for that of other people, the virtues of justice and beneficence; of which, the one restrains us from hurting, the other prompts us to promote that happiness. (1759 Part VI: conclusion 1)

Records indicate further that the historical Phillip aligned himself with the rise of enlightened liberalism in his time by insisting on equal rations for marines and convicts and other democratic gestures.[33] His style of government suggests allegiance to the tradition of contractual social theory so prominent in the period. Locke stipulated a century earlier that "the great end of men's entering into society" is "the enjoyment of their properties in peace and safety;"[34] the foundational premise of this society is "the preservation of society, and (as far as will consist with the public good) of every person in it" (1689: xi.134: 158). Legislation is sanctioned by "the consent of the society" (1689: xi.134: 158) and is "limited to the public good of the society" (1689: II.xi.135: 159). Moreover, by failing to call the assembly of representatives of the people (or parliament) into session, or exercising arbitrary power, a tyrant is not merely abusing his power but performing a "breach of trust" (1689: xix.222: 197).[35]

Nonetheless, there is no indication that the historical governor deliberately sought to implement the theories of Jean-Jacques Rousseau, while Wertenbaker's Phillip mentions Rousseau directly in the play (*Country* 18) and it is her Phillip who creates an analogy between the dynamics of a small republic and those of drama's back-stage teamwork.[36] In his *Second Discourse* (1755), Rousseau contested Hobbes' assertion that man is naturally aggressive, claiming instead that it is the capricious existence to which men are subjected in civilized society that stifles natural benevolence and forces them to compete with and contend against one another. In nature, animals are not inclined to attack others of the same species unless in self-defense or cases of extreme stress. At the same time, civilized man has lost his natural vigour; has grown "weak, timid and servile" (Rousseau 1755: 52) and his indulgence in unnecessary luxury has led to "deeper degeneracy." Warped civilization is responsible for the corruption of humanity, argues Rousseau: "man is weak when he is dependant, and he is his own master before he comes to be strong" (1755: 65). This seems to me an accurate description of the underlying claim of Wertenbaker's play and of the resulting effects Wertenbaker's Phillip expects his convict-play will have: the restoration of the convict's natural vigour while dissipating their hostility.

In *The Social Contract* (1762) Rousseau asserts, "the mere impulse of appetite is slavery, while obedience to a law which we prescribe to ourselves is liberty" (1762: 178). According to Rousseau, the community should be governed by serving "the general will" (which is the best interest of the collective body and not necessarily consensus among its individuals).[37] In this, at least, Hobbes, Locke, Smith, and Rousseau all agree—the best basis for securing cooperative government is a balance between altruistic idealism and practical self-service: the pursuit of personal gains which at the same time provide collective profits.

Effective government of the general will require wise legislation and wise leadership. Phillip provides this. Major Ross expects "insubordination, disobedience, revolution" (*Country* 23); Philip envisages a "contract" (*Country* 59) between himself and his subjects.[38] Consequently, Phillip believes that once the convicts are granted civil rights and are allowed to live independent and respectable lives, they will conform of their own accord to the greater good of society.[39]

In order to "rule over responsible human beings, not tyrannize over a group of animals," and against the prevalent penal theories of his times, Phillip proposes reform through "kindness" (*Country* 58–9). His chief kindness is to consider his post not to be that of a chief warden of a penal colony but of a leader of a reform project that will found a new democratic society. At great personal risk and despite the possibility of a mutiny (*Country* 59), Phillip remains a steadfast Sentimentalist, believing in the possibility of moral and social betterment.[40]

In *The Theory of Moral Sentiments* (1759) Smith acknowledges that our psychological makeup includes "malevolent and unsocial passions" such as anger and resentment. However, through subduing these passions by exercising others, "the benevolent and social affections" may triumph. This necessitates social institutions that encourage such moral civilization. Wertenbaker's play places drama at the forefront of such institutions. Perfection is not attainable, but we can and should aspire to "imperfect but attainable virtues" (1759 Part VII II.i.42).[41]

Our Country's Good demonstrates that, in addition to the invaluable personal advancement facilitated by drama, political gains may also be made by rehearsing a comedy. In the political climate of the late twentieth-century, such a claims were often deemed self-contradictory. For instance, Stephen Weeks draws parallels between Governor Phillip's behavior and that of the leaders of the new Virginian colony described in Stephen Greenblatt's famous essay "Invisible Bullets." Weeks argues that in both cases, testing a subversive hypothesis is the means by which the settlers "maintain their dominance" over their respective colonies, replicating their "old value system on a new continent" (Weeks 2000: 150). Weeks also claims that just like the Virginian viceroy, Thomas Harriot, ensured civil obedience by introducing products of European civilization such as religion and technology, so too Wertenbaker's Philip introduces the King's English to his natives (the convicts), thereby ensuring their submissiveness (151). This line of argument coheres with Ann Wilson's complaint that the occasion of the convict-production, the birthday of the king, produces a patriarchal image of England that reinforces imperialism (Wilson 1991: 31).[42]

Weeks and Wilson's claims reveal some confusion between the historical viceroy Arthur Phillip, Keneally's H. E. in the novel and Governor Phillip in the play, when the three ought to be kept distinct from one another. Their criticisms also suggest multiple misreadings of the play. Although it is true that, by teaching the convicts to speak Farquhar's "well balanced lines" Ralph, at Phillip's behest, is displacing their native tongue and replacing it with the language used by those in power, this can hardly be said to be a means of subjugation. The convicts, as we are expressly shown in Act I onboard the deportation ship, could not possibly be more subjugated than they already are. The fact that the convicts literally speak a different language from the officers only reinforces their subjugation. The complaint that Philip ingeniously contains the subversion he himself instigates by "recruiting" the convicts to his cause is equally shaky. Liz, writes Weeks, is made to submit to Phillip and exhibit complicity with "an ideology to which she had been unalterably opposed" (152). Similarly, Esther Beth Sullivan concludes, "the convicts willingly subjugate their futures to the will of their benevolent dictators and provide the basic day-to-day labor which is necessary to build the Empire" (Sullivan 1993: 143). She goes so far as to claim that the "good" theater that Wertenbaker presents is based upon the convicts learning to "deprioritize their complaints for the benefit of the 'small republic' which is theater" (144).

Steeped in Marxist politics and Foucauldian theory, these critics see the substructures of domination and manipulation where they should see Wertenbaker's play. Liz categorically does not join the old oppressive order but, rather, the new *liberal* order she discovers through Phillip's kindness. "The question of Liz" dramatizes Rousseau's claim that the difference between man and beast is not only the potential for emotional, intellectual, and spiritual advancement but in agency—in the application of free will: "it is in his consciousness of his liberty that the spirituality of his soul is displayed" (1755: 54). The moment that Liz realizes that she can participate, even monopolize the authorship of her own life story, is also the moment in which "the spirituality of her soul" is revealed. Moreover, though it is true that Liz is "recruited" and that she accepts that such recruitment entails "private sacrifices for the good of the whole" (*Country* 90), this is not a form of capitulation. On the contrary, "recruitment" is the very condition of her freedom.[43]

Smith argued that behavioral patterns and moral values are necessarily influenced by the company one keeps. As social creatures, we humans are naturally disposed to

> accommodate and to assimilate, as much as we can, our own sentiments, principles, and feelings, to those which we see fixed and rooted in the persons whom we are obliged to live and converse a great deal

with, is the cause of the contagious effects of both good and bad company. The man who associates chiefly with the wise and the virtuous, though he may not himself become either wise or virtuous, cannot help conceiving a certain respect at least for wisdom and virtue; and the man who associates chiefly with the profligate and the dissolute, though he may not himself become profligate and dissolute, must soon lose, at least, all his original abhorrence of profligacy and dissolution of manners. (1759 Part VI II.i.17)

This claim is best understood through attention to the final scene of *Our Country's Good*. In this scene, convict John Wisehammer expresses the wish to substitute Farquhar's prologue to *The Recruiting Officer* with a satirical prologue he has written himself. Despite admitting it to be very good, Ralph rejects the prologue on the grounds that "it's too—too political. It will be considered provocative" (*Country* 90). On the one hand, Wisehammer's feat of personal initiative, creativity, and literary merit marks the extent to which the convicts have been liberated from their previous shackles and provides an example, just as robust as the one Liz provides, of the success of Phillip's experiment. On the other hand, it has been argued that this scene constitutes a containment of subversion. I agree that, while Wertenbaker allows authority to be challenged during rehearsals, that the actual performance of *The Recruiting Officer*, which leaves out Wisehammer's prologue, contains part of that challenge. And yet, the expression "our country's good," which Wertenbaker chose as the title for the entire play, is taken from Wisehammer's prologue. This may be "another instance of the persistent irony that underlies even the moments that most strongly affirm the theater's progressive, redemptive power" (Weeks 152). But the issue of subversion—and thus its potential containment—is deliberately introduced by the prologue Wertenbaker herself writes for *Our Country's Good*.[44]

Historical records indicate that it was the epilogue that was written by a convict, not the prologue, though no record of the text survives. In *The Playmaker* the text Keneally writes for this epilogue is not subversive but is, rather, quite endearing. More importantly, Keneally's Ralph thinks it excellent and Wisehammer is not only allowed to end the performance with it, he is also assigned the delivery of Farquhar's opening prologue, which most of the audience (knowing no better) attribute to him.[45] Wertenbaker's text is the only one featuring satire and subversion. Furthermore, Wertenbaker's Sideway consoles Wisehammer by promising that his prologue can be used in "the Sideway Theater" (*Country* 90) that he intends to found when freed.[46] This suggests quite forcefully that Wertenbaker is not interested in suppressing subversion. Her interests lie elsewhere entirely.

As Ralph explains in the play, Wisehammer's sacrifice is precisely the kind of sacrifice individuals are called upon to make for the benefit of the community (*Country* 90). Thus, Wisehammer subordinates his personal desires to the "general will." This is not a form of regression but of advancement. His behavior evidences the ability to defer satisfaction and to exercise prudence—moral values promulgated by Smith.[47] As explained above, Rousseau holds that one of the conditions for the preservation of civic rights afforded by the rule of law, is the curtailment of personal liberty. "What man loses by the social contract is his natural liberty and an unlimited right to everything he tries to get and succeeds in getting; what he gains is civil liberty and the proprietorship of all he possesses" (1762: 178).[48]

Humans are social creatures who naturally seek to form communities. These communities, more often than not, consider the safety of the community more important than the personal liberty of its individuals. The desire for justice, security, and prosperity are often prioritized above complete freedom. As Isaiah Berlin explains in his *Two Concepts of Liberty* (1958), solidarity, equality, and fraternity should not be confused with liberty.[49] Moreover, unbridled personal liberty comes at a very heavy price, that of loneliness. To live among humans is to submit to a universally beneficial non-aggression pact and to hope and strive for a community that takes care of its own. Admittedly, this necessitates a certain restriction of individual liberty, but few people would forego the advantages that come with these restrictions. As Wisehamer himself admits in Act II.x: loneliness is "the worst" condition of all (*Country* 40).

The tremendous personal gains achieved in rehearsals do not have to be broadcast to the entire colony in order to be tangible and valuable, but the performance, on the other hand, must take account of its audience, in which there are objectors. Rehearsals lasted almost six months and have transformed all those who took part in them to a degree that will shape the rest of their lives. This process can neither be contained nor revoked. But the true test of the project is revealed in the convicts' understanding of civic responsibility. Wertenbaker makes this clear by ending *Our Country's Good* just before the performance of *The Recruiting Officer* begins. We already know that the collaborative, redemptive activity of production has been successful and we have been privy to its irrevocable process. It has served as a grand rehearsal for real life in a real republic.

To lament Liz, Dabby, or Wisehammer's loss of independence, or to suggest that their natural desire for self-determination is oppressed by a coercive political regime is to impose ideologies upon the convict's helpless loneliness. The alliances and friendships that are formed during the production of *The Recruiting Officer,* which allow Mary to call the actors a "family" (*Country* 88), constitute precisely that which they have longed for all their lives. The convict-actors are delivered from the misery of isolation by the warm embrace of communal life and form for themselves a supportive republic.

Further yet, the dynamic dramatized by Wertenbaker follows Smith's assertion that humans naturally aspire to social harmony brought on by the full recognition of their potential:

> Man naturally desires, not only to be loved, but to be lovely; or to be that thing which is the natural and proper object of love. He naturally dreads, not only to be hated, but to be hateful; or to be that thing which is the natural and proper object of hatred. He desires, not only praise, but praise–worthiness; or to be that thing which, though it should be praised by nobody, is, however, the natural and proper object of praise. He dreads, not only blame, but blame-worthiness; or to be that thing which, though it should be blamed by nobody, is, however, the natural and proper object of blame. (1759 Part III ii.1)

The "sanitized, rationalist vision of the Enlightenment" (Reddy 125), which later generations inherited, is a nineteenth century retroactive view of the preceding century, colored by the traumatic effects of the reign of terror in France.[50] The Enlightenment went hand in hand with a "cult of sensibility." The deconstruction of the mind-body binary seems to have been attempted, with substantial success, a number of times in our cultural history, but was always later stifled by a rationalist counter-reaction. *Our Country's Good* celebrates a point in time at which Sentimentalism was deemed rational—and suggests current audiences may see the value of such views for their own times.[51]

Drama can offer us a glimpse into a world beyond the claustrophobic, power-oriented ideologies of late twentieth-century theory, and beyond the idealization of personal and national autonomy that, more often than not, result in a sense of isolation. Wertenbaker attests that:

> I don't think you can leave the theater and go out and make a revolution...But I do think you can make people change, just a little, by

forcing them to question something, or by intriguing them, or giving them an image that remains with them. And that little change can lead to bigger changes.... (Chaillet 1988: 554)

Drama can initiate and facilitate positive change. Viewing a play and, even better, taking part in its production, convinces us of our ability to trust in embodied receptiveness and in one another. As Governor Philip explains, theater reminds people, "there is more to life than crime, punishment...We will laugh, we may be moved, we may even think a little" (*Country* 18).

More than Shakespeare and Stoppard together, Wertenbaker unashamedly defies suspicion and cynicism, demonstrating instead how we may create, maintain, and advance better forms of personal and communal existence than current paradigms often presuppose. The kind of social commitment dramatized in *Our Country's Good*, by joining humans together, acknowledges our natural propensity to "relatedness" (Haidt xii)—our need, as essential as sustenance, to form bonds with others. Wertenbaker's play looks back to eighteenth century theories and forward to the new era of the post-Postmodern. Restructuring our philosophical, political and literary theories so as to accommodate the fundamental structure of human cognition is simply acknowledging that it is time to anchor our pursuit for justice, knowledge, and happiness in our richest resource: our own bodies.

Chapter 4

"A Spiritual Dance:" Moisés Kaufman's *33 Variations*

When I have fears that I may cease to be
Before my pen has glean'd my teeming brain,
Before high-piled books, in charact'ry,
Hold like rich garments the full ripen'd grain;
[...]—then on the shore
Of the wide world I stand alone, and think
Till love and fame to nothingness do sink.

(John Keats 1818)

The protagonist of *33 Variations* is Dr. Katherine Brandt, is an elegant and respected musicologist in her late sixties.[1] Though her field of expertise has been Ludwig van Beethoven, she betrays no signs of romantic or Romantic inclinations. She is evidently devoted to her work, but her commitment is characterised by fierce interest and focus, rather than passion. Her brisk, restrained manner suggests she has always been efficient, and very much in control at all times. And this strategy has served her well, so far, at least in terms of her professional achievement. However, the play begins a few weeks after she discovers she has an incurable disease. The rapid deterioration of her health and the inescapable demands thrust upon her by her physical disintegration, force her to inhabit the body she hitherto almost ignored. The effect is not merely a re-evaluation of her life's choices but an overhaul of her relationships—professional and personal. The radical cognitive shift that occurs when she becomes conscious of herself as embodied, just at the inception of that body's dissolution, precipitates an existential reconfiguration.

Just as Shakespeare, in "Sonnet 18," promises his poem will provide his beloved with immortality; just as Stoppard's Joyce claims his work will "double that immortality" (*Travesties* 42, Chapter 2 of this book) so, in *33 Variations,* the characters of Beethoven and Katherine achieve immortality through their respective works. However, I shall be arguing that Kaufman's attitude to the necessarily finite nature of human existence also elucidates a condition Martin Heidegger terms "Being-toward-death" (1927: Division II.I, 235). One of the central ironies of *33 Variations* lies in that the most honest and most intriguing work of its protagonists is accomplished towards the very end of their lives, when they are fully conscious of their imminent demise. Like Keats, their need to have gleaned their "teeming brain" is not an attempt to stave off or defy their inevitable death, but a powerful motivating force.

In this chapter I suggest further that learning to trust the body, and learning from that body, do not cease when that body begins to fail. Quite the contrary. When illness hijacks one's body, reducing one to an observer of a seemingly independent process of annihilation, the deconstruction of the body may facilitate a reconstruction of the self. Giving birth to a new subject position can produce knowledge of a kind that could not, perhaps, be tapped by the healthy agent. As Einat Avrahami has argued, "it is the experience of illness as a process of learning that underscores the changed body as a source of knowledge" (Avrahami 2007: 4). It appears that before it decays, "the full ripen'd grain" can, if one is attuned to it, inspire a creative energy that both invites insights and reveals pathways for communicating them to others.

I. The Primary Cause: Creative Inspiration

The subtitle of *33 Variations* asserts that this is "a play in variation form." The play is not divided into scenes but into exactly thirty-three variations, emulating its chief intertext: Beethoven's composition. In music, variations begin with an initial core or "theme" material that is then repeated and/or elaborated upon in multiple altering forms, which may include changes in harmony, melody, counterpoint, rhythm, timbre and orchestration. Theme-and-variation form first emerged during the sixteenth century, but Beethoven's "33 Variations" was so innovative and powerful that it has been described by Alfred Brendel as "the greatest of all piano works" (Kinderman 1995: 211). Kaufmann's adaptation of the variation form to drama already, in itself, merges theme with technique. *33 Variations* thus continues Shakespeare's "mixed-mode" approach, and Stoppard's intertextual acrobatics, resonating in both theme and technique with many of the insights discussed in chapters 1 and 2, while, at the same time, offering a fresh angle from which to asses these insights. Both Beethoven's and Kaufman's 33 Variations, by delighting in various interlinking forms, extend the celebration of multiplicity and interdisciplinary cross-fertilization expressed throughout this book. In particular, this play celebrates life through confronting death. Alain Badiou and Nina Powers define death as "that whereby, beyond the derisory being-multiple of living individuals, the existence of life affirms itself. Every time that a living thing dies, what is silently spoken is: "I, life, exist"" (Badiou and Power 2002: 65). Kaufman's play suggests that the fact that death is the final variation of each life does not have to darken that life; it may even illuminate it, if we are, in Heidegger's sense, attuned to the possibilities this condition may precipitate.

Although we cannot report the experience of our own death, nor benefit from the reports of others, the termination of life remains a compelling topic for existential contemplation because we know that it is the final outcome of our existence. Attitudes to death and, more importantly, to dying, are quintessential to existential choice. In Heidegger's terminology, "attitudes" imply understanding "attunements." These are types of future-oriented awareness that also involve an emotional investment in "existential possibilities." Those modes of existential choice that adequately express and reveal the structure and possibilities of human existence are "authentic;" while those modes that disguise, ignore or misrepresent such possibilities are "inauthentic." As opposed to other animals, humans are aware that, in principle, they will die at some point: "Factically, one's own Da-sein is always already dying, that is, it is in a *being-toward-its-end*" (Heidegger 1927: 235). In the inauthentic condition, one "*knows*" about the certainty of death, and yet "*is*" not really certain about it" (238, italics in the original).

At the opening of the play, although she has recently been diagnosed with Amyotrophic Lateral Sclerosis (ALS), Katherine does not intend to change her lifestyle in any way. She is not yet ready to face the implications of her disease and is, quite consciously, evading them. Psychoanalysts would say she is "in denial;" Heidegger would describe her attitude as inauthentic. Despite her daughter Clara's protestations, Katherine plans to dive headlong into the research required for a new monograph. She sets out to investigate why Beethoven, already deaf, spent a substantial amount of energy in his last years writing thirty-three variations of a waltz written by Anton Diabelli. At the starting point of this investigation, Katherine explains that Beethoven, in 1819, "is only tackling major works. He has very little time left. And yet he chooses this mediocre waltz as his next project" (33V: "THEME": 9). She is not yet aware of the ironic connection to her own condition, which leaves her "very little time left," and yet she decides to begin an investigation into the very same waltz. She is trying to pursue her career as ambitiously as before and this research project is not embarked upon with any consciousness that it is her last "major work." She has not yet unpacked the significance of her "need to know" (33V: "THEME": 9) precisely this, rather than any other aspect of Beethoven scholarship.

History records that Anton Diabelli, music publisher and minor composer, approached a number of eminent contemporaneous composers, inviting them each to create a variation of a waltz he had written, to be published as a single, extended variations piece. Katherine assumes Diabelli's proposed project is a means of self-advancement since, she reasons, his "less than stellar waltz" (33V: "THEME": 6) would be thus honored by the most talented composers of the day, placing him on a par with them; it would also be lucrative for him as the publisher. But, more than anything else, it would not only "immortalize" his waltz (33V: "THEME": 6) but himself.[2] What intrigues her, however, is the reason for which Beethoven would stoop to partake in such an enterprise. The initial impetus for her study, then, is less Beethoven's final achievement than its moment of origin—like the dream that inspired "The Rime of the Ancient Mariner," or the drug-fevered trance that, allegedly, inspired "Kubla Khan."[3]

The play begins and ends with a correlative of the musical theme that serves as a backbone for any musical variations piece. While the pianist (downstage) plays the Diabelli theme that inspired Beethoven's "33 Variations," the word "THEME" is also projected in large capital letters onto the stage-screen. The opening lines of the play are Beethoven's, spoken by Katherine:

> Let us begin with the primary cause of things.
> Let us begin with how something came about.
> Why it came about in that particular way
> And became what it is. (33V: "THEME":1)

After a short pause, Katherine adds, "For me, it begins in Vienna, in 1819." Through this condensed opening statement, Kaufmann informs the audience that Katherine's is a subjective interpretation of events, predicated on the assumptions that the beginning of the process she seeks to research can be determined and, moreover, fixed to a particular place and time; that the unfolding particularities of the journey that commences can be traced; and that the end product—"what it is"—can be delineated. All these assumptions are, of course, highly contestable. As the play progresses, Katherine is forced to acknowledge the fluidity of time, of meaning, and of being. Gradually, she discovers that "what it is" is open-ended, like Diabelli's short waltz which "had so much [...] to offer" Beethoven (33V: "JOYFUL SILENCE": 77). In the context of the play, this piece "change[s] everything" (33V: "THEME": 1) for Beethoven, as it does for Katherine, impressing upon her the recognition that the only constant in the universe is change: everything is in perpetual flux.[4]

In his introductory note, Kaufman states that he has "chosen to explore this story from a fictional perspective. Thus, this play is not a reconstruction of a historical event; rather, it's a series of variations on a moment in a life." Following in kind, this chapter does not present historical accounts that may verify or challenge Kaufman's imaginative response to the historical core of the tale, but focuses upon the implications and possibilities suggested by Katherine's evolving interpretations of it and the impact this has upon her understanding. For instance, Katherine's initial data include the biography of Beethoven written by Beethoven's secretary, Anton Schindler. In Bonn, she soon discovers Schindler's biography evidences many "inaccuracies" (33V: "THE DISCOVERY": 79). Thus, even the first hand or "historical" accounts of this reconstruction/interpretation are themselves partial and fallible, and so possibly misleading. In other words, her project will require a great deal of conjecture, and there will be little data from which unequivocal answers may be ascertained. Indeed, when Katherine first arrives at the Beethoven Archives in Bonn, Dr. Gertie Kinderman, keeper of the records, confesses she is uncertain whether the archival material could be of any use at all to Katherine's particular interest, since it is "really a question of inspiration." (33V "THE SKETCHES – PART 1": 28).

Beethoven's contemporary, William Wordsworth, famously announced in his *Preface to Lyrical Ballads* that

> poetry is the spontaneous overflow of powerful feelings: it takes its origin from emotion recollected in tranquillity: the emotion is contemplated till by a species of reaction the tranquillity gradually disappears, and an emotion, kindred to that which was before the subject

of contemplation, is gradually produced, and does itself actually exist in the mind. In this mood, successful composition generally begins.
(*Preface*: 273)

Katherine's attempt to locate the moment Beethoven's "successful composition" began requires her to enter into a particular "mood" that may tap into what Gertie calls "an unadulterated first impulse" (33V: "THE SKETCHES – PART 1": 29). This process can neither be forced nor rushed; it depends not upon an accurate knowledge of dates and facts, nor of compositional rules but, instead, upon engaging empathetically with the artist himself, what Wordsworth calls "a being possessed of more than usual organic sensibility" (*Preface*: 265). Only a physical and emotional immersion in Beethoven's life and works may hope to resonate with—rather than uncover—his inspiration.

At the opening of the play, Katherine is wholly unequipped for such a task. In her prologue, she conjures Vienna in 1819: "The effects of the French revolution are still being felt all over Europe and the ideas of freedom and equality are galvanizing people's minds" (33V: "THEME": 5). What Katherine does not say is that the failure of the revolution has already led to stricter censorship and policing; that Byron and Shelley, whom she mentions, are both already in exile; that Keats has already contracted tuberculosis and that, although Goethe and Hugo publish books that year, the Romantic revolution is already passed its heyday. The moment she chooses as the moment the Variations "began" is not an isolated moment; it is influenced by the preceding century's political upheavals, by the Romantic movement, by the current climate at that particular place and time—Vienna 1819—and by the constellation of creative artists in Vienna at the time, notably Schubert, Liszt, Czerny and, of course, Beethoven. What captures Katherine's "imagination" (33V: "THEME": 5) is the question of what captures Beethoven's imagination—a Romantic theme indeed. But can it be captured?

When, in the play, Diabelli first invites Beethoven to contribute a variation to his project, Schindler replies, "his mind is completely occupied with other commissions." Though this is Schindler's construction, and is intended as a means of politely declining the invitation, thereby extricating his master from a frivolous project, it is nonetheless telling. First because, as the play unfolds, Beethoven's mind becomes obsessively "occupied" with this very waltz. Second, because this commission is not freely undertaken. "What it is," as Katherine would put it, is a kind of hostile "occupation" of the composer, a kind of possession, from which he will not be exorcised until he has drawn out all the variations it may generate.

When Gertie first leads Katherine into the multitude of towering shelves filled with sketchbooks and books in the Beethoven Archives, Kaufman notes that they should seem to "*go on forever*" (33V: "THE SKETCHES – PART 1": 29). Already on entering this subterranean treasure vault, the stage set suggests the infinity of time. These sketchbooks are the remnants of a man long gone—a testimony to his compositional process, his "original inspiration," the "initial instinct," and perhaps most importantly, the physical link between the past and the present. Full engagement with these relics will entail a leap of the imagination, a transcending of boundaries.

When Gertie opens the first book, known as the "Wittgenstein Sketchbook," she explains it consists of "forty-three leaves of "Honig" paper" (33V "THE SKETCHES – PART 1": 30). Honig is of course honey, and the image of the honey combined with "leaves" resounds with Wordsworth's "organic" imagery. It also conjures the ancient mystical symbolism of man as a beehive and of (spiritual) knowledge as honey.[5] The implication is that this research will lead to spiritual rewards of a kind that far transcend what Katherine imagines she has bargained for. Additionally, an analogy is created between Beethoven, Katherine, and Wittgenstein himself, who continued to write to the very end, though dying of prostate cancer. Like Beethoven and Katherine, Wittgenstein's Being-toward-death was characterized by a spurt of creative energy. Interestingly, his final philosophical investigation, *Remarks on Color*, was inspired by Goethe, tying him further into the Romantic theme of this play, while inviting a further analogy between the immeasurable impact of Wittgenstein's and Goethe's respective contributions to philosophy and literature, and Beethoven's impact on music. In particular, all three thinkers are renowned for their fearless originality. Among their many innovations, Goethe's *Theory of Colors*, and Wittgenstein's investigations of it, transformed conceptions of color thereafter. Similarly, though Mozart, Handel, Hayden, Schubert, and Bach, all wrote variation pieces before Beethoven, and Beethoven himself wrote some variations before the "33 Variations" on Diabelli's waltz, the approach, technique and power of his 33 Variations changed the genre thereafter; Chopin, Brahms, and Elgar were already writing in the wake of Beethoven's genius. Beethoven dismantled the traditional form, replacing it with an entirely new, and flexible structure.

Such connections within connections, variations upon variations, and attention to creative thinking, set the scene for the kind of knowledge that Katherine, who is initially rather rigid, will have to learn during the last few months of her life. While she is able to appreciate genius, she is not presented as a genius herself, nor does she suppose herself to possess such qualities.

However, Kaufman's play dramatizes the stages by which Katherine internalises the potential inherent in the claims, made by Romantics and Existentialists alike, regarding the degrees of authenticity with which each individual may respond to possibilities and create new ones.

At the opening of the play, however, she is not yet aware that her inflexibility is a drawback. Instead, although Katherine's journey to Bonn is undertaken for the purpose of research, her main motivation seems to be flight, both from her disease and from her fraught relationship with her only daughter, Clara. She thinks very highly of her daughter's natural gifts but she is frustrated and disappointed by what she interprets as Clara's lack of drive or direction: "Clara was always piercingly observant and original in her thinking. [...] But her ability to function in the world, has always been, not deficient, per se, but rather uneven" (33V: "HERE BE DRAGONS": 65). Because Clara is so talented, and yet refuses to stick at any particular profession for long, it seems to Katherine she will "always be mediocre at everything" (33V: "RESEARCH": 14). Katherine's view of Clara is not unlike her view of Diabelli's "mediocre" achievement, treating both as "a second rate waltz" (33V: "MORPHINE": 102). She is equally mistaken about both because she is trapped by a narrow definition of value.

While Schindler worries that Beethoven is wasting [his] time on the Variations, when he should be writing his Ninth Symphony; Katherine considers anything other than her work on the Variations a waste of time. Clara has tremendous respect for her mother's research yet, nonetheless, cannot reconcile herself to being totally shut out of Katherine's last few months. Clara's efforts to insinuate herself into her mother's presence and affection achieve only limited success until Clara is able to make a substantial contribution to Katherine's work. Piercing the invisible wall between them is accomplished when Clara redefines herself in her mother's eyes through impacting her research. On the day Clara leads Katherine to view Diablelli's waltz and Beethoven's obsession with it from a different perspective, Katherine is also finally able to accept and respect her daughter's life-choices.

II. Embodied Resonance, Tactile Therapy and Authenticity

Though Clara and Katherine finally connect in the realm of Katherine's work, this connection builds upon foundations laid down in Bonn over the previous weeks. Kaufman's play suggests that it is the body that grounds the spirit. While exploring the sketches for Variation #3, Katherine is captivated by Beethoven's transparency:

> These three notes C, A, B flat.
> Repeated over and over.
> He's pausing to think.
> A lesser composer would have erased that passage, or changed those
> bars, but not him.
> He wants you to see his moment of trepidation, of doubt.
> (33V: "THE SKETCHES – PART 1": 34)

Katherine, not entirely aware yet of her own trepidation, is becoming conscious of having embarked upon a journey of a kind she has not yet attempted. This meditation upon the process of (creative) choices is followed immediately by attunement to physical reality. Katherine notices a stain on the manuscript paper. She assumes it is wine. No, explains Gertie, "it's probably soup. He loved soup. [. . . the sketch-books] are not only a record of his compositional process, they are also a record of his daily diet" (33V: "THE SKETCHES – PART 1": 34). The short intermission that follows, in which Beethoven shouts at his housekeeper for preparing a "putrid, fetid, rancid, rotting trough of swill" (35) adds a humorous dimension to the scene that provokes some comic relief, but it also carries profound implications. We are not allowed to forget that Beethoven's genius was bound up with his human body. Neither he nor Katherine can ignore the needs, desires, and failings of their bodies. The soup not only leaves an indelible mark on the manuscript pages, imposing its presence upon the composition, but becomes an inseparable part of the puzzle, just as Katherine's failing body will be instrumental in her own inquiry.

The very next scene, Variation: "CLASSICAL MUSIC," is indeed a variation on the same theme. Clara and Mike, out on their first date, are attending a concert at which, significantly, a pianist plays Variation #8. Kaufman's audience is privy to the character's racing thoughts, pre-recorded like a filmic voice-over, but the only action that takes place on stage is hand movements. Mike reaches out to Clara, hesitates and withdraws, and finally dares himself to clasp Clara's hand. She responds in kind. He exalts: "Best, Concert Ever" (37). The forceful impact of a physical gesture is brought to the forefront. Bodies communicate. This clasping of hands equals a contract—hands have been shaken, bodies have touched, souls are entwined.

Two scenes later, the hand theme is continued, with a variation of course. Gertie and Katherine are waiting for a train. Gertie notices Katherine's hand is limp, "Oh it's nothing, nothing," protests Katherine (33V: "BASEBALL": 42). Katherine's habitual denial of her disease, and the running theme of nothing/something in the play, come to a brief halt when she finds herself confessing to Gertie that she has ALS and, at the same moment, discovers Gertie already knows this, because she has personal experience of caring for an aunt who died of the same disease five years earlier. At this point, the bond between the two women is cemented. Katherine knows Gertie knows not merely that she is ill but how the illness can be expected to proceed, and for what eventualities Katherine must prepare; and she knows Gertie will be truthful and direct: no euphemisms, no false hope.

The presentation of the potentialities of embodied resonance in *33 Variations* also elicits empathetic resonance in its viewers. Bruce McConachie argues that "Our ability to empathize with the experience of others through mirroring is the cognitive hook that impels spectator interest in the activities of actor/characters and engages us in the enfolding narrative of the play" (McConachie 2008: 18). Though empathy is not itself an emotion, he reminds us, "it readily leads viewers to emotional engagements. In addition to experiencing unconsciously the six basic emotions, spectators often gain a conscious awareness of their emotional commitments, which encourage them to form sympathetic or antipathetic attachments to certain actor/characters" (65).[6]

Kaufman's development of the physical dimension of his character's experience, and of the play's preoccupation with embodiment, reaches a peak in Variation "EXAM," in which Katherine's body is exposed to the audience. She has to take off her top for an X-ray examination. Her nakedness symbolises the extent to which she is stripped bare; no defences, physical or cultural, can protect her from the ordeal she must undergo. The respectable professor becomes terminal patient, or even lab rat. But the power of this scene resides it its directness. Though spectators are aware that, within the context of the play, Katherine is alone in a private room and is, thus, unconscious of any external gaze, their positioning as fourth-wall audience, in full view of her naked body, renders them voyeurs. At this moment, our privileged status as audience—enjoying the play without having to take part in its painful proceedings—becomes compromised. Although one of the pulls of the theatre, as of literature and cinema, is that it offers intimate and comprehensive access to the minds and hearts of characters in a way that rarely occurs in life, spectators are still likely to feel discomfort when gazing thus upon Katherine's abasement.[7] Objectively speaking, spectators know that the doctors do not intend to humble but to treat her. Yet these doctors are, significantly, absent, while the audience's presence in this moment of fear and dejection is very real. We become witnesses, and are thus implicated in Katherine's humiliation.

In addition to eliciting empathy, sympathy, and pity, this variation hurls viewers into an unmediated confrontation with the experience Sartre theorised in terms of the phenomenology of shame.[8] In the Broadway production, this mixture of feelings was intensified, at least for me, by the fact that Katherine was played by Jane Fonda. Fonda is over seventy. While part of me was struck by her beauty and dignity as a woman, and her courage as an actress, I felt that staring at her nakedness was somehow a breach of decency, of trust. Moreover, in that production, Fonda was seated on a cold, metallic table, which made the examination seem all the more threatening. Her feet did not reach the ground, making her seem small and vulnerable.

During "THE EXAM," Kaufman's stage directions require Katherine to turn left and right. Not only is she half-naked and alone, but also the flashes of light seem invasive: almost as if the machine is torturing her. Moreover, being a musicologist, Katherine is very sensitive to sound. Kaufman describes the sound of the machine as a "brutal" force that "bruises her" (33V: 58) and, in performance, when it becomes apparent that she finds this experience harrowing, a further analogy is established between her pain and that of Beethoven who, in the previous variation, experiences excruciating ringing in his ears as he slowly advances towards deafness. The experience of pain is so acute that no intellectual strength may override it, and both characters' existential condition is reduced to the physical awareness and mental distress that accompany this invasion of their bodies.

Just at this moment, however, Katherine hallucinates Beethoven. He comes in, silently, and sits on the gurney behind her. Katherine slowly leans back until she finds his back and leans on him, her head resting on his back. The image of this silent act is one of the most memorable of the play. Kauafman's direction spells out his intended implication: "she finds a modicum of peace and comfort in the subject of her obsession" (33V: "THE EXAM": 58). But it also further connects the two as suffering bodies. Suffering cannot be eliminated, but it may, perhaps, become meaningful, as illness makes for kinder, more sympathetic bodies. Kaufman thus reinforces and extends the confidence in bodily knowledge advanced by each of the plays studied in this book.

Interestingly, it is soon after their bodies touch that Katherine finds the will to face her condition authentically. As Heidegger explains:

> Authentic being-toward-death signifies an existentiell [sic] possibility of Da-sein. The ontic potentiality-of-being must in its turn be onto-logically possible. [. . .] Da-sein is constituted by disclosedness, that is, by attuned understanding. *Authentic* being-toward-death can*not evade* its ownmost non-relational possibility or *cover* it *over* in this flight and *reinterpret* it for the common sense of the they. [. . . Being-toward-death is] a being toward an eminent possibility of Da-sein itself. (239–241; italics in original)

Though Heidegger does not discuss the function of bodily-awareness as a means to achieving the courage required to face one's Being-toward-death, and though Kaufman makes no explicit references to Heidegger, it seems to me that Kaufman's play directs his audience to see the connection. Once Katherine becomes truly one with what Avrahami terms "the idiosyncratic validity and veracity of concretely situated, embodied experience" (Avrahami 2007: 14) and, crucially, once she is able to, quite literally, recognize that inter-corporeal communication is a source of comfort and assistance, she is also able to resume control of her life.

She instructs Gertie and Clara as to exactly what arrangements she wishes to secure. First, she implores, "If I cannot make myself understood I want to be given morphine and left to die" (33V: "MORPHINE": 100). Second, she wants Gertie, rather than Clara, to decide when this is the case. "I am doing you a favor," she tells her daughter, "so that you won't have to make these decisions" (100). She asks Mike to obtain the narcotic, and Gertie to administer it. She cannot predict when she will need it, but she is in full control of what will happen when she does. However, she cannot anticipate the degrees of change she will undergo before that moment comes; neither can she anticipate that this change will be precipitated not through conscious, systematic choice, but though involuntary bodily involvement.

Kaufman does not provide Katherine with much of a personal history and so the audience cannot know for certain, but we may surmise from her demeanour that her attitude to her body is based upon a legacy of North American WASP culture, born of the Puritan tradition, with its fear of sensuality and its no-nonsense work ethic. Her denial of her disease is but an extension of her life-long denial of her physicality, and her conscious reliance upon practical and logical considerations over either sensual or sentimental ones. Like Leontes in *The Winter's Tale*, Katherine has been denying herself both the comfort and solace that come with intimacy, and the knowledge that it provides.

But people need to touch and be touched. Tiffany Field, Director of the Touch Research Institute, in Miami, Florida, has asserted that many people in society today may actually be suffering from a shortage of tactile stimulation, a phenomenon she evocatively terms "touch hunger." Our skin contains receptors that can elicit emotional (sometimes referred to as affective or hedonic) responses. As Field points out, "Touch is ten times stronger than verbal or emotional contact, and it affects damned near everything we do. No other sense can arouse you like touch...We forget that touch is not only basic to our species, but the key to it" (Field 2001: 57).[9]

As her condition worsens, Katherine's physical deterioration undermines her strident independence and allows her to submit to the mollifying effects of interdependence. In an attempt to alleviate her pain, and slow down her debilitation, Mike not only begins to practice physiotherapy upon her, he teaches Clara how to do so too. Mike's role in the play is, from his first appearance, that of a healer. But he is not a miracle worker. Rather, he is patient and caring; he listens, and he is well versed in the language of embodied receptiveness. At first, neither Clara nor Katherine want to touch one another, they are so unpractised in expressing physical tenderness. But with Mike's guidance, treatment becomes a collaborative effort and, through finally forcing Clara and Katherine to touch, mother and daughter move past their psychological resistance, just as Liz does when the piece of wood is pronounced her fan (Chapter 3). Initially, Mike has to model the movements and Clara must learn through imitation. Gradually, however, the awkward mechanical imitation is transfigured into its better self: simulation that elicits empathetic engagement.[10]

Einat Avrahami contends that "the crisis of serious illness generates extreme, new experiences and sensations that can break down
the habits of a lifetime" (2007: 162). Kaufman seems particularly
interested to dramatize the specific effect bodily contact may have in
this context. Touch has been a part of the healing process in many
civilizations and cultures throughout the centuries. However, recent
clinical studies show that "it is possible to experience moments of
pleasure in the midst of being a severely ill patient at an ICU and,
through this experience also gain hope" (Henricson et al. 2009:
323). Many hospitals incorporate reflexology or other forms of
touch-therapy into their care program, as patients often benefit from
human warmth and consideration, even through a hug or a pat on
the cheek.[11]

The practice of "tactile touch therapy," specifically, has been
shown by Henricson and her colleagues to be extremely effective.
Tactile touch involves slow stroking with firm pressure, mainly
performed with the flat of the hand with fingers close together[12]
and even when administered behind a curtain in a crowded ICU,
has been described by patients as creating an "imagined room of
togetherness" which provides "the opportunity to focus on oneself"
in an environment of calm, caring security, dispersing "nightmares,
thoughts and worries about illness" as well as "disturbance from
other patients and/or staff during the tactile touch" (Henricson et
al. 325). Moreover, Henricson asserts that being "connected to oneself" through "being in touch with one's body and mind" elicits not
only a sense of harmony and peace but a sensation that "time and
being in togetherness are intertwined" (327). For a patient such
as Katherine, whose deterioration is terrifyingly swift, a session of
gentle, "tactile touch" could very feasibly provide an oasis of calm,
during which time is stopped, slowness may be enjoyed. Most pertinent to the arguments presented in this book, Henricson and her
colleagues show that the feeling of togetherness fostered by touch of
this kind "contributed to feelings of being privileged, which meant
to be treated with respect, asked for consent" and, further, pro-
moted "feelings of security and reciprocal trust, which contributed
to a possibility to take control over the situation" (327, underlining
in original).

In *33 Variations*, Mike's instructions draw Katherine and Clara
out of their habitual antagonism and into a place of mutual trust.
This affects the very core of their being. Kaufman represents this
through their breathing. The breathing exercises Mike prescribes

realign mother and daughter, yielding "a momentary truce" (33V: "PHYSICAL THERAPY": 74). This metonymic invocation symbolizes their physical and imaginative identification, and points to a connection through powerful emotional resonance and solidarity that, at least in part, fends off the potential objectification, marginalization, and isolation of the terminal patient, creating a community that shoulders her pain. A moment later, Katharine is doubling up with laughter; a symptom Mike calls "emotional incontinence" (33V: 75). Productive as the physical communication may be, it still involves one body that is speeding towards death.

Controlling one's breath is, of course, central to Eastern traditions of meditation. Thus, in addition to the obvious physiological effects of an unobstructed and energizing flow of oxygen, this act also symbolizes a new state of expansive readiness, or availability of body and spirit. Malekin and Yarrow claim that the meditative breath prepares one for a state of openness to regeneration and change, by "expanding the inner space, adjusting the spinal column and causing the whole body to come into a condition of restful balance" (Malekin and Yarrow 1997: 136). Even more poignant, they describe this state as "beginning to function in tune," that is, in harmony with oneself and the world, a "liberation from the shackles of habit" (137). This final construction echoes Kaufman's implied meanings and his very linguistic choices. The symmetry created by Katherine and Clara's synchronized breathing, the calm introspection and shared embodied resonance dramatized in this variation, suggest coordination: both taking control and letting go, empowering the self and reaching out to others.

Physical therapy cannot allay all doubts and fears; it cannot override the swift progression of the disease or its inevitable outcome. But it can alleviate Katherine's private struggle and ground her spirit in the very real knowledge of the embracing presence of love surrounding her. Humans are social animals. We can survive many adversities; we may even survive alone. But we are much happier when we establish healthy, lasting bonds of friendship, love, and trust with other fellow humans. One cannot describe Katherine as happy. But the power of the "relatedness," which psychologist Jonathan Haidt locates as the most profound conduit to happiness (Haidt 2006: xii), cannot be underestimated.[13] Katherine's newfound closeness to her daughter, her unexpectedly intimate friendship with Gertie, her trust in Mike— these connective threads, proof of dependable companionship, profoundly influence her state of mind and her courage to contend with the difficulties ahead. "Yes," explains Mike, "that's one of the benefits of ALS. It forces intimacy" (33V: "INTIMACY": 104).

When Katherine's limbs begin to fail, she makes use of a stick, then a walking frame. When her tongue withers, Mike gets her an "augmentative speech device." Technology compensates, for a while, for her physical handicaps. It also advances empathetic communication. Mike explains to Clara that, if she is herself immobile while she learns how to use the device, it will give her "a closer sense" of what her mother needs to know (33V: "THE DISCOVERY": 82). Moreover, it is through this machine that Mike tells Clara for the first time that he loves her. Kaufman thereby demonstrates Clark's theory of "cognitive scaffolding" (Clark 1998: 274), which extends our cognitive potential through cooperation between brain ("wetwear"), body ("hardwear"), and environmental aids ("widewear").[14]

After declaring his love, Mike tells Clara he could tolerate his own body deteriorating as long as he had shared some of his life with her (33V: "CHEESEBURGER": 85). Clara melts at this inept attempt at romancing and then confesses she worries that, when Katherine dies, she will lose her external-gauge, the moderating force that keeps her in check: "how do I know I won't totally fuck up my life?" (33V: "INTIMACY": 105). Mike answers: "You know you said when you look at your mother you see grace? [...] every time I look at you that's exactly what I see. Grace" (ibid). It is time Clara acknowledged that she and her mother are far more alike than either likes to admit; that while she must necessarily be a continuation of her mother's genes, she can choose how she wishes to direct that continuation; that she has the grace to do so in a unique and creative fashion. In existential terms, she can harness her facticity to serve and advance her authentic creative fashioning of herself. Finally, she can also admit that Mike is not merely a fit substitute for her mother, but the catalyst for a new variation of herself. Not surprisingly, her response is "let's have sex [...] I just want to feel healthy" (105–6). Acknowledgement of the entirety of the self, exercising creative flexibility, enjoying physical contact and fostering effective communication with others—all these equal health. Defined as such, health is a condition Cavell and Spolsky would certainly deem "good enough."

But it does not occur to the lovers that this equation may still apply to Katherine. Gertie, on the other hand, does not forget that, sick as she is, Katherine is still a physical being. She suggests they hire Katherine a masseur. "Do you think a woman with A.L.S. has no sexual appetite?" (33V: "CAFETERIA FOOD": 93). The matter-of-fact tone of her delivery is sincere. Just as Beethoven liked his soup, so

Katherine still has her own desires. Pain often marks our individuation. Effective as our mirror-resonance mechanisms may be in generating motor equivalence, and powerful as our drive to sympathy may be, we can never fully experience the pain of another. Touch, however, "provides us with an often-overlooked channel of communication" and plays "an important role in governing our emotional wellbeing" (Gallace and Spence 2010: 247). Furthermore, the effects of touch are temporary. One needs to be touched at regular intervals. At no stage in life does one overcome the longing for intimacy.[15] Further still, touch often elicits memories from previous instances in which we enjoyed physical contact (Henricson 327). As Paula M. Niedenthal et al. have argued, "when a person's body enters into a particular state, this constitutes a retrieval cue of conceptual knowledge...In turn, other cognitive processes, such as categorization, evolution, and memory, are affected...[and] biases other cognitive operations towards states consistent with that emotion" (Niedenthal 2005: 40).[16]

Due to her experience of illness and pain, Katherine is forced to reconstitute and redefine herself. As Manuella Consonni claims, the radical nature of such experiences "does not cancel knowledge but redeploys and sharpens it [...] giving rise to an entirely different way of perceiving the world and comprehending the events that take place in it" (Consonni 2010: 3).[17] As Katherine's epistemological boundaries shift, her cognitive scope, bound to her failing body, unveils a new typology of knowledge. While the experience of illness can never be fully conveyed in language, it can, in some situations, such as those dramatized in this play, override its exclusionary manifestations and create new channels for communication that were previously blocked.

This is in great measure due to the radical (and often irrevocable) changes wrought by illness. Haidt explains that nerve cells respond vigorously to new stimuli, but gradually they "habituate," firing less to stimuli to which they have become accustomed. "It is change that contains vital information, not steady status" (Haidt 2006: 86). Change revitalizes. Although the changes Katherine undergoes are almost all unwelcome, they are also, ironically, vehicles for pleasurable sensations too. The disruption of her life by the advent of her disease, the anguish that accompanies her confrontation with her finite existence, the process of a protracted and gradual Being-toward-death, are accompanied by the thrill of immersion in her research, by the thrill of new challenges, and by the curative effects of her physical contact with her daughter. Together these lead to breakthroughs in both her work and her personal life.

III. Time and Transfiguration

From the moment she rests her back against Beethoven's on the gurney in the MRI lab, the two timeframes of the play—Beethoven's and Katherine's—begin to merge. As their bodies begin to malfunction, and modalities begin to compensate for one another (such as reading lips and imagining music instead of hearing) more and more scenes present a space-time[18] continuum, in which several characters from different timeframes are present on stage simultaneously, having separate yet closely interlinked conversations; often saying the exact same words at the same time. One of these is "I need more time" (33V: "SEPTET": 61). Time is relative, the speed of its passing subjective, but as indicated by Keats in the epigraph to this chapter, its urgency is shared. Being, as Heidegger argued, is always already Being-in-time. In variation "SEPTET," which completes Act I, Gertie speaks to Katherine in Bonn, in 2008; Mike speaks to Clara in New York, in 2008; Schindler speaks to Beethoven in Austria, in 1822:

> GERTIE AND MIKE
> You have to slow down.
>
> KATEHRINE, CLARA, BEETHOVEN
> Time is scarce.
>
> DIABLELLI AND CLARA
> I can't wait any longer.
>
> BEETHOVEN AND KATHERINE
> I have so much to do.
>
> SCHINDLER, MIKE, GERTIE, DIBAELLI
> Please. (33V: "SEPTET": 63)

As the empathetic connections between the characters strengthen, so the geographical and temporal gaps between them dissolve.

> MIKE
> Listen to me. You have an opportunity here.
>
> BEETHOVEN
> I must not lose this opportunity.
>
> KATHERINE
> This is my last opportunity.
>
> CLARA
> This is my last opportunity.
>
> BEETHOVEN AND KATHERINE
> I must have the chance to finish the work.

At one point, Gertie literally takes a notebook from Dibaelli's hands and reads it in the archives, two hundred years later (33V: "THE CONVERSATION NOTEBOOKS": 69).

Kaufman's melting of space-time barriers, and his dramatization of physical contact between characters inhabiting different time-frames, presents a view of temporality and of human connectivity that may be more than just dramatic effect. Many leading physicists today are convinced that a multiverse system is not merely hypothetical. As physics professor and cosmologist Max Tegmark asserts, "it is becoming increasingly clear that multiverse models grounded in modern physics can in fact be empirically testable, predictive and falsifiable. [...] the key question is not whether there is a multiverse [...] but rather how many levels it has" (Tegmark 2003: 1).[19] In *Postmodern Science Fiction and Temporal Imagination*, Elana Gomel argues that the traditional view of time as a linear sequence of past, present and future is not only too narrow to encompass the complex *timeshapes* of temporality, it ignores the inroads made into time-analysis by evolutionary theory, quantum mechanics, cosmology, cyberspace, globalization, and the resurgence of religious fundamentalism. "Time and space are physical, not just mental and cultural, aspects of the universe," asserts Gomel. But, she continues, space-time is "inaccessible to us except through the filter of narrative" (Gomel 2010: 7). "There is no such thing as 'natural,' 'private,' or 'psychological' time that predates its narrative emplotment" (8). As Paul Ricoeur argues in *Time and Narrative* (1983), narrative creates an intelligible form for existence:

> between the activity of narrating a story and the temporal character of human experience there exists a correlation that is not merely accidental but that presents a transcultural form of necessity. *To put it another way, time becomes human to the extent that it is articulated through a narrative mode, and narrative attains its full meaning when it becomes a condition of temporal existence.*" (Vol 1 52, emphasis in original)

Beethoven and Katherine's narrative "emplotment" transcends space-time, physically and spiritually.

Then, at the opening of Act II, Katherine addresses the audience directly. Viewers may assume they are, for her, the imagined audience attending the conference at which she plans to deliver her paper on the Variations, but this direct appeal instantiates further spatiotemporal fluidity. Moreover, her address concerns transfiguration, "not the Christian variation but the abstract idea": "transforming one thing into something better. Moving from the banal to the exalted" (33V: "HERE BE DRAGONS": 64). Alfred Brendel claims that, in Beethoven's Variations,

> The theme has ceased to reign over its unruly offspring. Rather, the variations decide what the theme may have to offer them. Instead of being confirmed, adorned and glorified, it is improved, parodied, ridiculed, disclaimed, transfigured, mourned, stamped out and finally uplifted. (Brendel 2001: 114)

In this variation, Katherine considers, for the first time, the possibility that Beethoven is not merely mocking Diabelli but transfiguring his waltz. In that case, she muses, the Variations are not an exercise in "making something out of nothing" but, instead, a study in "transforming the waltz into its better self" (33V: "HERE BE DRAGONS": 64).

In the given conditions of our universe, "making something out of nothing" is impossible. The world is comprised of various composites made up of a limited set of components. Individual humans and the world at large are made of the same atoms, combined in multiple forms that produce various effects—variations on a theme.[20] If there is, as many Romantics argued, and Clark has recently further asserted, a continual symbiotic relationship between brain-in-body and world, and if, as quantum physicists now suppose, time is not necessarily linear but a complex web, then Kaufman's play dramatizes a fictional instance of a probable scenario—a collapse of empirical boundaries that does not collapse the distinctions between the various entities/phenomena, yet leads to communicative breakthroughs. Perhaps "nothing will come of nothing" (*King Lear*) but something is always becoming something.

Katherine, however, is well aware that this something may not necessarily be an improvement. At an early stage in the play she already acknowledges that

> My motor neurons are deteriorating rapidly. Every day my muscles are receiving fewer and fewer signals from my brain, so they are atrophying.
> But the best part of this is that my brain remains untouched by the illness! So that I am able to fully experience the process by which my body is becoming but a flaccid carcass.
> Transfiguration indeed. (33V: "HERE BE DRAGONS": 64)

Ironically, she will be transfigured, but not in the way she envisages at this point. She is even able to consider the possibility that "perhaps children ought to be the way in which we transfigure" but, she adds, "my own daughter is a mystery to me. Children! HERE BE DRAGONS!" (33V: "HERE BE DRAGONS": 65).

Clara soon after explains that English mapmakers in the sixteenth century placed the phrase "here be dragons" at the edges of their known world. "They meant to imply that a) well, there are dragons there, and b) that venturing into those regions was a risky proposition" (33V: "HERE BE DRAGONS": 66). Katherine sees in her daughter not merely alien territory but a "risky proposition" at the edges of her "known world." Clara represents a world apart, a parallel universe, in which the rules are so different Katherine cannot fathom them. Beethoven calls his manuscript pages his "children" (33V: "BEAUTY": 91) and the audience is well aware that Katherine's life energies go into her work, her professional child. But Clara is no dragon. To the contrary, she plays the part of St. George by trying to slay the dragon that guards her mother, self-entrapped in her ivory tower. Since the only route into Katherine's universe traverses her professional life, Clara will have to make a substantial contribution to Katherine's research if she hopes to penetrate her mother's battlements.

Katherine's first discovery is that it was Schindler who started the legend that Beethoven hated Diablelli's waltz. This implies that "we truly have no idea what Beethoven thought" (33V: "THE DISCOVERY": 80). After nine months in Bonn, corresponding to the nine months of gestation, or Beethoven's Ninth Symphony—all Katherine seems to have gained is uncertainty. However, in contrast to Leontes in *The Winter's Tale*, this realization does not cause her to lose her bearings. Katherine had suspected that Beethoven sought to elevate himself through mocking Diabelli. By the time this hypothesis is questioned, she has already learned the value of flexibility, and tests another: what if he did it for the money? (33V: "THE DISCOVERY": 80). This hypothesis is soon discarded, as it proves so discordant with what she knows of Beethoven's character.[21] A third hypothesis is then tested: what if he did it to outnumber Bach's 32 "Goldberg Variations"? But this too does not seem likely.[22]

Then, one evening, Clara comes into the kitchen, absent mindedly humming Diabelli's waltz. Katherine is amazed. It has never occurred to her that someone may like the waltz for itself and she asks Clara to explain what it is that she likes about it. Clara remarks simply: "it has a pretty melody. It has a nice rhythm. [...] You can feel the rhythm" (33V: "A PEACE OFFERING": 109). Feeling had not been factored into Katherine's rigorous research. Once Gertie starts singing and tapping out the rhythm of the Variation, pounding the table and stomping her feet, it also dawns on her that this waltz "was a beer hall waltz, not a concert hall waltz" (33V: "A PEACE OFFERING": 109). Physical engagement with the music reveals a different set of interpretive possibilities. There can be no external validation for any of their hypotheses; they cannot know for certain what Beethoven intended and, even if they did, this would not cancel out alternative interpretations of the piece. But *feeling* the rhythm of the music suggests an interpretation that *feels* intuitively right. Gertie is gracious enough to attribute the breakthrough to Clara, exclaiming: "You've made a musical discovery!" At this moment the floodgates open—all three women in that kitchen experience a gestalt—reminding us of the Wittgenstein sketchbook. Katherine's excitement is so great she begins to choke.

Clara's instinctive delight in the "pretty" melody of Diabelli's waltz leads Katherine to surmise that Beethoven's objective is not grandiose. This is a beer-hall waltz, turned into multiple other dances and culminating in a gentle minuet; it pays homage to community, freedom, laughter and the curative powers of music. Gleaning the playful jollity from this piece becomes his greatest inspiration, analogous to celebrating what is left of life itself. Either Beethoven found the original waltz "commonplace" (33V: "THEME": 7), as Schindler recorded, and then discovered it was richer than he had anticipated or, as Clara leads Katherine to hypothesize by the end of the play, he found it rich precisely because it was commonplace—because its theme was that of Everyman.

This hypothesis seems to me corroborated by the prevalent contemporaneous interest in the common, a linking of Wordsworth's leach-gatherer with Beethoven's Biergarten. Moreover, it is known that Goethe held Byron in the highest regard. By 1823, when Beethoven completed the Variations, he may well have also been acquainted with *Don Juan*. Perhaps he was familiar with the ironic narrator's impudent assertion that:

> Man, being reasonable, must get drunk;
> The best of life is but intoxication:
> Glory, the grape, love, gold in these are sunk
> The hopes of all men, and every nation;

Without their sap, how branchless were the trunk
Of Life's strange tree, so fruitful on occasion: (DJ 2:178 lines
   1425–1431)

Moreover, Beethoven's Ninth Symphony can be seen as further proof
of this theory, as it is more closely affiliated with the Variations than
Schindler or Katherine suppose. Although this is not discussed in the
play, one may assume that Katherine, a Beethoven scholar, would know
that the inspiration for the Ninth Symphony is Friedrich Schiller's "Ode
To Joy" (German: "Ode an die Freude," 1785), which celebrates the
ideal of unity in brotherhood of all mankind. Although it was written
before the French Revolution, at the height of Republican idealism, it
remained of profound and lasting influence despite the failure of the
revolution, and was set to music by Beethoven as the final movement of
his greatest symphony.[23] Like the Variations, the Ninth Symphony was
a protracted project that occupied Beethoven for many years.[24] This
suggests that both the Symphony and the Variations aim to convey a
similar theme: happiness captured in varied instances, joyous celebration of multiplicity. Moreover, Beethoven combines theme with form
by disregarding the customary rules of symphony composition. In addition to the tonal, orchestral music, he added choral passages, both for
four soloists and a choir, an unprecedented variation on the traditional
form. His composition emphasizes his creative use of convention, his
interest in harmonizing various human voices, and in celebrating joy.

The play, however, focuses at this point upon Beethoven's growing
sense of urgency:

> I must NOT be a human being.
> I must not be for myself alone.
> […] The music will free people from all the misery and all the indig-
>   nities that shackle other human beings. (33V: "NOT A HUMAN
>   BEING": 111)

When Schindler objects to this heresy (or megalomania), Beethoven
retorts: "you putrid appendix! […] How could you, being so vulgar, appreciate anything that's not vulgar?" (33V: "NOT A HUMAN
BEING": 112). There is a value to the lofty and the sublime but,
Beethoven is implying, there is also refinement in detecting the sublime in the ordinary, something in (supposed) nothing.

The theme of something/nothing in the play recurs often, mark-
ing a further Existential undercurrent.[25] The variations form is

extended to encompass the life choices of the main characters, and the final movement sides with an Existential view, which focuses on subjective human experience rather than objective truths, and the human struggle with (or against) the apparent meaninglessness of life. For the Existentialist, there is no predetermined truth, no right way to do something, no specific something for which to aspire, but an active self-creation motivated by free will (limited as it may be by facticity): making choices, being accountable for those choices, and taking responsibility for the consequences. Kaufman's Beethoven declares, "if I show respect for a person, it will be because that person earned my respect with his deeds" (33V: "ACCIDENTS OF FATE": 55). Initially, Katherine misjudges Clara, Gertie, and Mike, but learns to respect each in turn by acknowledging their deeds. It is not that audiences are called upon to see either Clara or Katherine as an ideal, Kierkegaard's *knight of faith* or Nietzsche's *Übermensch*, but we are invited to see their different variations on the theme of existence, and the productive dialogue these variations produce by the end of the play, as a model path to authenticity as described above by Heidegger.

Moreover, Clara undergoes a transfiguration no less profound than her mother's. In Act I, Clara explains that "I love doing something for a few years, getting good at it and moving on. For me that's a life better lived" (33V: "DANCING": 50). For years, her mother misunderstands this as dilettantism. Katherine's swift movement towards death, ironically, allows her to appreciate Clara's choices, different as these are from her own. Clara, she finally sees, has always been naturally attuned to the variation form. She not only expresses herself in multiple, evolving, creative forms, she enjoys each variation. Until this point in her life it was her mother's exacting and censoring disapproval that prevented her from bursting "Joy's grape against [her] palate fine" (Keats, "Ode on Melancholy 1820)—from celebrating the great Nietzschean "Yea." When Mike enters her life, just as her mother's dominant presence evolves into a new variation, Clara is finally able to let her spirit soar.

IV. Being-toward-death:

By 1822, Diabelli already has fifty variations, written by other eminent composers. Though Beethoven could continue beyond his thirty-three, even he understands that neither Dibaelli's nor his own time can be extended infinitely. When Beethoven gets to Variation #32, he seeks a variation that "exists far from the theme" in a "foreign key." His process mirrors Katherine's sojourn in Germany, her own foreign key. This variation prepares for closing, it "forc[es] us towards resolution" (33V: "FUGUE": 97). Katherine and Beethoven are working now on the same theme: "how does one begin to let go?" (33V: "INTIMACY": 106). When he lets go, he completes the Variations; when she lets go, she allows Clara into her heart, which also resolves her academic quest.

The concrete, situated body can be interpreted in many ways, but its ontological presence cannot be denied, nor can its ultimate dissolution. However, the process of illness and of individual responses to it can be an indispensable source of knowledge, "stressing the experience of terminal illness as an embodied process of learning to live with extreme physiological, and not merely social, constraints" (Avrahami 12). Grappling with her unruly body forces Katherine to abandon previously set structures. The material self can no longer accommodate its past forms but must constitute a new somatic identity and a new conception of self. But this does not eradicate her anxiety; until she confronts her fears head-on, she will not be freed of their oppressive presence.

Towards the end of Act II Katherine is once again wheeled into an MRI machine, while a live projection of her face appears on the large screen onstage, filmed from above, closely monitoring her horror. Once again, the examination room seems invasive, loud, tortuous. Then, Katherine draws once more upon Beethoven to free her from her indignities, singing "kyrie eleison" (33V: "NOT A HUMAN BEING": 114). Kaufman has Katherine, Clara, Schindler, and Diabelli all sing this portion of Beethoven's choral symphony in four-part harmony. His directions stipulate: "It is a meditative and prayerful moment in which they have left the reality of their surroundings and search for comfort in the beauty of music. They are all in need of a merciful G_d" (33V: "NOT A HUMAN BEING": 115).[26]

In the next variation, Beethoven appears before Katherine: "Oh no," she exclaims, "I was hoping I wouldn't hallucinate. It doesn't look good in a scholar" (33V: "LIMBO": 116). This statement suggests that their previous meeting on the gurney was a theatrical metaphor; it was Kaufman's means of expressing Katherine's dependence upon Beethoven, a reflection of her unconscious experience. In this variation, however, they talk freely. Like Catherine in *Wuthering Heights*, Beethoven tells Katherine he has fled heaven,[27] together with all the great composers of all times: "the angelic music made me wish I was still deaf" (33V: "LIMBO": 116). He recalls that it took him twenty-five years to finally lose his hearing completely. The oscillation between hope and despair was unbearable. When, at long last, all hope was gone, he actually felt relieved. "I would never hope again. And lo and behold, I was able to create music that would never have been possible had I been in the world of the hearing" (33V: "LIMBO": 117). Katherine gains validity through this confirmation of a paper she wrote arguing just that; and she needs her projection of Beethoven to tell her what she already knows: that it is "time to stop struggling" (33V: "LIMBO": 118). Katherine will finish her monograph just as she has learned to ask her daughter to help her scratch her own nose (33V: "BREAKFAST": 122), just as they are finally able to cry together, just as she has understood Mike is the man for her daughter. Resolution is complete.

One of the quintessential elements of drama requires the characters to learn, adapt and change in time.[28] If they do not, the play is probably a tragedy. If they do, even if the play ends in the protagonist's death, it is no tragedy. As deeply as Clara and the audience may mourn the loss of both Beethoven and Katherine, their deaths are accompanied by a sense of satisfying completeness. Death is insurmountable, loss is agonizing, but the life that precedes death is the central focus of this play, and this book. Moreover, the experience of death is largely determined by each individual's attitude to, and preparedness for, its eventual arrival. Neither Beethoven nor Katherine, nor Clara, Mike, or Gertie are taken by surprise. They all accept, in their own ways, that time is simply up, and that it is the state of Being-towards-death that counts most in this ultimate transfiguration.

As Heidegger asserts, authentic awareness of the ineluctable allows one to view the possibilities clearly, and to choose among the possible responses to one's facticity; the limitations within which we may exercise (free) will:

> Becoming free for one's own death in anticipation frees one from one's lostness in chance possibilities urging themselves upon us, so that the factical possibilities lying before the possibility not-to-be-bypassed can first be authentically understood and chosen (243–244).

> Being-toward-death is essentially Angst; [...not in the sense of fear or cowardice, but in the Existential sense of facing the possibility in] *passionate anxious **freedom toward death** which is free of the illusion of the they, factical, and certain of itself.* (245; italics and bold in original)

That is why, though Clara is the one who delivers Katherine's paper at the conference, since her mother is already dead, the play nonetheless ends on a triumphal note. Clara reads out Katherine's words:

> I propose that Beethoven [...] was showing us what lies in every moment of the waltz.[...] Variation form allows Beethoven to do the miraculous and slow down time, to pierce the waltz and enter the minutia that life, in its haste, robs us of [...] it is a way to reclaim all that is fleeting. (33V: "VARIATION #33": 123–124)

When Katherine first arrives in Bonn, Gertie introduces Beethoven's sketchbooks as "survivors" (33V: "THE SKETCHES – PART 1": 29). Though Katherine could not possibly survive her illness, her work will survive her. She has conquered the disease by making it the very tool via which she unpacks the mystery of her research project. Her illness, her physical decay, gives birth to a survival testimony—a book by a woman on the verge of death about a man on the verge of death—both of whom galvanize their imminent demise to produce inspirational work. This does not diminish the enormity of Clara's loss. Many in the audience will have experienced losing a parent and some will have lost both. The triumph of the play's conclusion does not negate our sympathy but transfigures it into a final variation. Beethoven's Variation #33, a gentle minuet, becomes in Kaufman's play "a graceful dance" (33V: "VARIATION #33": 124) to mirror the grace of all the play's characters.

V. A Spiritual Dance

Schindler records that, after a protracted illness from which Beethoven emerged in 1822 with a completed masterpiece—the last movement of The Ninth Symphoney—he still claimed that he would, from then on, endeavor to surpass everything he's ever done before (33V: "THE CONVERSATION NOTEBOOKS": 70). The fact that then, after a three-year break, he was drawn back to the Variations, suggests this piece is, to him, a surpassing of all his previous accomplishments. And the play ends as it began—with Beethoven's lines about the primary cause. We are reminded of Nietzsche's theory of "eternal recurrence," yet seem free to also perceive progress not mere repetition because, as the pianist plays Variation #33, all the characters begin to dance ritualistically, slowly joining hands to form a circle. Katherine enters the circle as well. Then Beethoven and Katherine are left alone on stage, as if having met in heaven, or a preferred musician's limbo; they can now finally "begin their discussion in earnest" (33V: "VARIATION #33": 126).

It is apt that the play should end with a dance, the physical enactment of Beethoven's musical inspiration. Engaging with the melody and rhythm of the music is both a form of receptiveness, of admitting influence and, at the same time, an active participation. Embodied experience, translated into dance moves, particularly those that require a partner, connotes not merely inhabiting the body but an expressive, harmonic and shared activity. It is also the physical manifestation of all the play's transfigurations, and places Beethoven as master of them all. As Kaufman's Beethoven declares: "It is impossible to express new ideas using old forms. When I am done with this set of variations, I will have revolutionized what we now understand to be variation form" (33V: "JOYFUL SILENCE": 77). By doing so, by transforming the very format of the variation paradigm, Beethoven not only instantiates his own genius but speaks the language of God: "I am an instrument of G_d! I am Bacchus who creates the most glorious wine for mankind and makes them spiritually drunken!" (33V: "NOT A HUMAN BEING": 111).

The creative endeavor in which the characters and audience have been immersed the whole play is now declared to draw its inspiration from God. Seeing the inspired artist as an extension of God-the-creator is a recurrent Romantic theme. It expresses a longing to be one with the universe and chime with its wealth of curative and (re)generative energies. Schiller opens his poem with the exclamation: "Joy, beautiful spark of the gods" (L1), connecting jubilation with divinity. Beethoven's reference to Bacchus looks forward to Nietzsche, half a century later, who saw the liberating joy of spontaneous, uninhibited, freedom best reflected in "the Dionysiac art of music" (1872 16: 76). It also resounds with multiple Romantic texts, not least among them Coleridge's "Frost at Midnight" (1798):

> [...] so shalt thou see and hear
> The lovely shapes and sounds intelligible
> Of that eternal language, which thy God
> Utters, who from eternity doth teach
> Himself in all, and all things in himself.
> Great Universal teacher! He shall mould
> Thy spirit, and by giving make it ask.(L58–64)

The most profound effect of opening oneself to these teachings is not to secure answers but to make one "ask." Knowledgeable as Katherine was at the opening of the play, she knew this argument intellectually but did not live it. Just as she knew she was eventually to die, but was not yet living an authentic Being-toward-death. It is her engagement with Beethoven's Variations, as filtered through her illness and its consequences, rather than her academic investigations, that leads her to fully comprehend the meaning of asking.[29]

The dialogue between Existentialism and Romanticism in this play does not determine its religious orientation, since neither school is tied to a particular faith. Nietzsche, the immoralist, was famously critical of the Western monotheist religions but his Zarathustra draws upon Eastern traditions. Heidegger did not characterize Da-sein in relation to the possibility of an after life, only in relation to our ontological existence in this world, but Kierkegaard and Jaspers were not only believers but also Christian theologians. Similarly, Wordsworth and Coleridge were both Anglicans, becoming more and more conservative as they aged, while Shelley was an outspoken atheist. Nonetheless, Shelley was committed to "the spirit of Intellectual Beauty," which seems to me close to the position Kaufman implies in *33 Variations*. The marked spiritual dimension of this play does not advocate any particular religion so much as a view of divinity-in-man-and-nature as the greatest source of inspiration.[30] As Schiller wrote: "joy all creatures drink / At nature's bosom" (L25–26).[31]

The Romantics saw perception as intrinsically active—a constant interaction between internal and external, between individual mind and nature. Beethoven's contemporary, William Wordsworth, wrote of

> A balance, an ennobling interchange
> Of action from without and from within;
> The excellence, pure function and best power
> Both of the object seen, and eye that sees.(*Prelude* XIII)

The sentiment of the final dance of Kaufman's play takes us back to the Romantic context of Beethoven's composition. In "The Aeolian Harp" (1796) Coleridge sees his poetry as an extension and passionate distilling of the "the one life within us and abroad" (L16). Man, nature, divinity and inspiration combine to achieve transcendence:

> And what if all of animated nature
> Be but organic harps diversely framed,
> That tremble into thought, as o'er them sweeps

Plastic and vast, one intellectual breeze,
At once the Soul of each, and God of all? (L 44–48)

In Coleridge's poem, the harp[32] represents the organic interplay between art (the lyre), the natural world that is inspired by the divine spirit (the wind) and the poet's creative mind. The correspondence with Beethoven's project is strengthened with every movement of Kaufman's play. Just as Coleridge's open window signifies receptiveness to "the one life,"[33] so Beethoven's variations project celebrates infinite possibility, the wealth and abundance germinating in apprehension of "the one life" or, in Schiller's phrase, "the great circle" (L21).[34]

Since the movement of the play is so closely modeled on Beethoven's, Kaufman may seem somewhat self-congratulatory when he has Katherine describe the last variation as a "spiritual dance" exhibiting "beautiful symmetry" in its design (33V: "VARIATION #33": 124). It is difficult to be both subtle and transparent, and Kaufman evidently opted for the latter. His continually evolving analogies, though true to the variation form, are at times a little too "symmetrical"; and he has been criticized for "canned sentimental dialogue about self-knowledge and self-acceptance" (Brantley 2009). But, like Wertenbaker before him, Kaufman is an unabashed paladin of sentiment. *33 Variations*, like *Our Country's Good* and *The Winter's Tale*, expresses confidence in the curative potential of uninhibited emotional communication. Moreover, the play's effusive emotionality is entirely in keeping with its Romantic contexts and intertexts. It also serves Kaufman's dramatic agenda well. The more spectators feel emotionally involved the more rewarding the experience of the play becomes. Kaufman deserves to congratulate himself for having, with sensitivity and sensibility, caused his audience to simulate the very cadence of the piece, undergoing a kind of transfiguration themselves, and emerging with an overwhelmingly satisfying experience of hope and trust.[35]

Many excellent plays, particularly those deliberately dramatizing alienation, isolation and nihilism (from *Hamlet* via Brecht and Beckett to Stoppard's *Rosencrantz and Guildenstern are Dead*) affect the viewer by challenging, shocking, disturbing, depressing. *33 Variations*, however, is remarkably elevating. As Malekin and Yarrow have asserted:

> If the essential spiritual function of narrative is to locate and activate the impulse to narrative—telling the story of meaning—the fundamental of drama is to enact and embody that story. [...] drama works

with the text of rich semiosis, across all channels of reception and via all the senses tuned to their full range from subtle to gross. (126)

Maynard Solomon likens Beethoven's "33 Variations" to an ascent: "Upward motion is present in virtually every variation". By dividing the work so that each subset of variations ends with a slow variation (# 8, 14, 20, 24, 29–31, and finally 33), argues Solomon, Beethoven's creation becomes an increasingly extreme and rarefied journey, "not merely from here to there but from here to higher" (Soloman 2003: 189). This movement echoes Hiadt's theory of elevation. Divinity, he argues, is a conception characteristic of the moral dimension of the human cognitive system: "the human mind simply *does* perceive divinity and sacredness, whether or not God exists" (Haidt 2006: 184). The sense of spiritual uplifting, the "glowing feeling" experienced by humans as a result participating in various religious rites, or by doing—or even witnessing—selfless good deeds and compassion, is a specific kind of emotion (with attendant physical properties, such as dilation in the chest), which Haidt terms "elevation" (195). This emotion creates a sense of calm well-being, hope and brotherhood, and inspires us to be virtuous ourselves. Mark Johnson also holds that human spirituality is embodied (Johnson 2007: 14) but, in his view, the spiritual dimension of life is best defined as *horizontal* rather than *vertical transcendence* (281). In other words, we are inextricably linked to our finite, physical selves, but we can go beyond that self and connect with

> a broader human and more-than-human ongoing process in which change, creativity, and growth of meaning are possible. Faith thus becomes faith in the possibility of genuine, positive transformation that increases richness of meaning, harmony among species, and flourishing, not just at the human level, but in the world as an on going creative development. Hope is the commitment to the possibility of realizing some of this growth—not in some final eschatological transformation of the world, but rather locally in our day to day struggles and joys. (281)

The result of either conception of embodied spirituality is the *feeling* of elevation. "Elevation may fill people with feelings of love, trust, and openness, making them more receptive to new relationships" (Haidt 2006: 198). This seems to me to be precisely what Beethoven aims to achieve through his music, and what Kaufman aims to inspire through his play.

This book begins by considering Shakespeare's demand that we awake our faith in the power of bodies in drama; it ends with

Kaufman's suggestion that not only is the body not antithetical to spirituality, it may be its very source. *33 Variations* does not propagate any established religious creed so much as spirituality in a broader sense, a certain degree and quality of awareness deeply embedded in our physical bodies. Unexplained as this process remains, matter gives rise to consciousness and, for lack of a less laden term, an indefinable force that may be termed spiritual energy, or the "one life."[36] This force, or motion, or Chi, or spirit, at the same time separate from any space-time location or functional limits, is channeled through and emanates from living bodies. It is responsible for transfiguring matter into life or, rather, it is that very transfiguration. Our multiple means of interacting with our environments—from physical architecture and sensations, via logic, inference, intuition, imagination, memory, empathy, emotional contagion, linguistic scope, and sympathy—also allow for elevation, inspiration, love, and trust. Learning to trust our bodies connotes reaching towards "the one life" and its manifold variations.

Conclusion

The Mind is its own place, and of itself can make a heaven of hell, a hell of heaven.

(*Paradise Lost* I.254–55)

Generosity, humanity, kindness, compassion, mutual friendship and esteem, all the social and benevolent affections, when expressed in the countenance or behaviour, even towards those who are not peculiarly connected with ourselves, please the indifferent spectator upon almost every occasion

(Smith, 1759 Part I II.iv.1)

Traditionally it has been claimed that evidence gained through empathy is epistemologically suspect as it does not have a truth-value. And yet, as I have been arguing throughout this book, humans tend to trust empathy instinctively. Empathy is an automatic mechanism of direct identification; the emotions it evokes are transmitted to the observer without requiring the mediation of theoretical inference; it is pre-conscious, pre-linguistic and appears to be one of the most basic of human inclinations, facilitated by our in-born mirror-matching mechanisms of simulation.

Nonetheless, simulation is not sufficient to interpret all inter-subjective encounters. As suggested throughout this book, basic emotional responses appear to be universal and we are able to decode them automatically. Complex (emotional) responses, however, require analytical, theoretical, and discursive forms of assessment, which can be culture-specific and difficult to translate. They are also, thus, open to greater degrees of potential error.[1] For empathetic interpretation to be creditable, it must rest secure upon the rationality required to differentiate good from bad inferences. Understanding requires a weighing up of both empathetic and theoretical kinds of evidence. As Henderson and Horgan assert, "we do well epistemically to employ

simulation and theoretical modelling as complementary processes—
and to employ hybrid processes" (Henderson and Horgan 2000:
130). Acknowledgment of the productive interplay between embodied receptiveness and analytical, linguistic assessment creates the possibility for knowledge the kind of knowledge Cavell and Spolsky term
"good enough." Any account of truth must, therefore, be freed of
"the myth of objectivism" (Lakoff and Johnson 1980: 160); truth is
"experiential" (175). There is no one Truth yet, as Johnson asserts,
there are "plenty of human truths," by which he means knowledge
that arises from the context of human embodied interaction. "Finite,
fallible, human truth is all the truth that we have, and all we need"
(Johnson 2007: 80).

The threat of radical skepticism, which often breeds an image of
the individual as trapped in solipsistic isolation, may be mitigated
through acknowledging that we do not engender ourselves—we are,
necessarily, part of multiple and various contexts: biological, cultural,
and emotional. Chapter 1 of this book demonstrates both how natural it is to doubt and how we may learn to trust; not in order to trade
painful truths for comfortable compromises, but as a means to those
very truths. Our minds exist in the context of our bodies, which exist
in the multiple contexts of other mind-bodies, communities, enmities, and alliances. In Chapter 2, Stoppard's inter(con)textual drama
provides further insight into the cultural-linguistic aspect of this
interconnectedness in art and politics, personal, and public identities.
In Chapter 3, Wertenbaker dramatizes the advantages of informed
and comprehensive understanding of extended community, in the
possibility of healing damaged bodies and psyches, and in the transformative powers of dramatic performance. And, finally, in Chapter
4, Kaufman suggests that it is never too late to learn from and to trust
in our bodies. Acknowledging our bodies allows us to truly inhabit
and thereby also transcended the divisions between individual bodies in space-time, facilitating effective communication (with ourselves
and with others), elevation, inspiration, love, and trust.

Since throughout this book I argue repeatedly that embodied
receptiveness facilitates greater understanding and trust, it is important to acknowledge that the same communication channels may also
be abused. Warren Poland has rightly pointed out that empathy is not
synonymous with sympathy, and should not be confused (as it often
is) with a general disposition to sociability.

> [C]onverting empathy from a form of perceiving into [a generic term
> for] interpersonal posture of warmth and goodness denies the many

ways empathetic perception can be used hatefully. The con man, the demagogue, the exploiter, and the sadist all function best when their empathetic skills are sharp. Indeed, the effectiveness of a sadist's cruelty is directly related to the capacity for empathy, to the ability to sense what will hurt most. (Poland 2007: 89)

It seems that our biological predispositions do not always predispose us to benevolence. In an article I published last year, I examine how Stephen Jeffreys's *The Libertine* (1994) and Lawrence Dunmore's film adaptation of Jeffreys's play (2004) provoke aversion in an effort to recruit the audience against the main protagonist: John Wilmot, the Second Earl of Rochester (1647–80).[2] This recruitment is conducted through an onslaught upon the senses of the audience; hijacking the viewer's moral judgments by accessing preconscious bodily mechanisms. The very basis of this project is sophisticated attunement to embodied receptiveness, yet its powerful effects signal the possible dangers our embodied receptiveness facilitates.

And yet, as Chapter 3 of this book demonstrates, simulation, motor equivalence, and empathy can be recruited for positive purposes—con men can be converted into actors, sadists into sympathetic republicans. The consciousness of the positive powers of empathy creates a sense of solidarity, of community—of shared interactive possibilities. Tying empathy to sympathy renders it liable to emotional and intellectual persuasion but, if we develop confidence in embodied receptiveness, such persuasion does not render empathy unreliable so much as a powerful humanizing force. While past generations were persuaded to neglect, even shun, the evidence of the senses, I hope this book serves to (re)instate embodied evidence at the top of the pyramid of our considerations: as the first (but by no means the only) essential component of our legitimate decision-making processes.

In fact, Roy Sorensen has proposed that empathy not only depends upon but also creates greater similarity between minds. Empathy "shapes minds in a way that makes them better suited to the exercise of this simulation technique" (Sorensen 1998: 75). While empathy exploits pre-existing similarities, sympathy forges new ones. This belief has political implications: "the revelation that we are even more mentally than physically alike shortens the step from self-respect to other-respect…our common humanity becomes morally relevant, not just self-congratulatory specieism" (78). Sorensen goes so far as to claim that our beliefs or desires may vary due to personal circumstances, but our makeup is identical: "to understand just one brain is to understand the organ for the whole species" (78).

If increasing psychic kinship promotes better understanding, sympathy and tolerance then, as I have been arguing here, dramatic performance, through tapping into our embodied empathic capacities, can be instrumental in defying radical skepticism. The very act of sitting in a theater and understanding oneself to have similar emotions to the rest of the audience already creates a sense of community. Dramatists do not need to be persuaded of this truth. But by applying evidence from multiple interdisciplinary fields ranging from biology, psychology, neuroscience, philosophy, and of course a range of performances, this study presents drama as able to provide us with tangible, effective, and lasting means with which we may encourage trust. Trust does not provide guarantees to absolute truth, if such a thing even exists. You may find that your trust was misplaced. That is a risk each one of us takes daily. But neither is trust merely a form of gambling. My hope is that you, dear reader, through reading this book, will have gained the confidence to forgo the embarrassed shrug of the shoulders that excuses your (seemingly naïve) decision, and feel instead justified when reaching an informed decision to trust.

Notes

Introduction

1. Krueger et al. show that "Conditional trust selectively activated the ventral tegmental area [of the brain], a region linked to the evaluation of expected and realized reward, whereas unconditional trust selectively activated the septal area, a region linked to social attachment behavior. The interplay of these neural systems supports reciprocal exchange that operates beyond the immediate spheres of kinship, one of the distinguishing features of the human species" (Krueger et al. 2007: 3).

2. Dr. David Servan-Schreiber has written extensively about forms of therapy that engage the body by accessing our physiology and emotions, without involving conscious, linguistic processes.

3. It will become apparent shortly that trusting plays does not connote expecting them to be "realistic" or covey a reliable mirror-image of the world. The many functions of fiction include responses to, extensions, complications, and illumination of reality, and creative experiments that are in no way tied to "reality." But we may trust in the powerful potential of drama to illustrate, elucidate, and engage us fully—accessing pre-conscious mechanisms as well as conscious thought.

4. Because this article has not yet been published it has no designated pages. It does, however, have numbered lines that I reference here.

5. For instance, Cromwell and Panksepp warn against conceptions of the brain as primarily a "computational device" (56) at the expense of incorporating recently supported "integrative functions that include dynamic neural networking that constructs organismic coherence and brain–body communication" (163–164). Similarly Bradford and Caramazza (2008) and Hickock (2009) object to unwarranted claims for either the motor-sensory aspects of cognition or their relation to intention-recognition.

6. Important "countercurrents to dualistic subordination of body to mind ran through the corpus of classical Greek and Hellenistic philosophical and medical traditions" (Bono 1997: 178). However,

both Western philosophy and the Church establishment shunned the role of emotion in knowledge acquisition. Moreover, while scientists studied the physical body, they too held that emotion was not to be trusted in the laboratory (Damasio 1999: 39). This prejudice continued well into the twentieth century, despite the extensive study of emotions conducted by Charles Darwin, William James, and Sigmund Freud at the end of the nineteenth century and beginning of the twentieth. Today, however, neuroscientists and cognitive theorists alike are aware that body and mind are two inseparable parts of a single living organism and are, by and large, interested in the evolutionary patterns that characterize this integrated whole (Damasio 1999: 40).

7. Haidt hypothesizes that "the frontal cortex is the seat of reason: it is Plato's charioteer; St. Paul's Spirit. And it has taken over control, though not perfectly, from the more primitive limbic system–Plato's bad horse, St.Paul's flesh. We can call this explanation the Promethean script of human evolution, after the character in Greek mythology who stole fire from the gods and gave it to humans" (Haidt 2006: 10).

8. I am aware of the fact that, because "embodied cognition" has sometimes been misunderstood to imply a reductionist view of cognition as entirely and solely generated by motor systems, it has created some opposition. Thus, Mahon and Caramazza's suggested "alternative" to the misguided notion of "embodied cognition" is, in fact, precisely the holistic view of interconnected networks propagated by this book from within the embodied cognition school.

9. For a review of this history see Gregory Hickock (2009).

10. Evidence obtained primarily through electroencephalography (EEG) and functional magnetic resonance imaging (fMRI), which provides information about regional cerebral blood flow and enables the analysis of neural activity, suggests that the human mirror system stems from activity in the inferior parietal lobe, inferior frontal gyres (including Broca's area), and superior temporal sulcus (STS) (Rizzolatti and Craighero 2004). For a detailed summary of the most important stages of this extensive research (traversing many countries, laboratories, and research-teams) see Agnew 2007.

11. For instance, cells in the STS (superior temporal sulcus)—at least in macaque monkeys—respond to a wide range of actions in a manner that appears more sophisticated than that found in MNs. STS cells, however, do not have motor properties (they do not appear to fire during action execution). Interestingly, the region of inferior parietal cortex that contains mirror neurons (PF) and which projects to F5, receives input from the STS (Rizzolatti and Craighero 2004).

12. When, for instance, a monkey hears a peanut being broken open, "local CDZs collect information about sensory input, and feed these

to a non-local CDZ that records the coincident information about the sound, sight and feel of this action. The CDZ does not hold all the details of the information; rather, it contains the potential to retroactivate the separate auditory, visual, tactile and motor sites, and thus reconstitute the original distributed set of memories and information" (Damasio 2008: 168). This implies that either MNs themselves are audiovisual or, at least, connect to long-term memories of previous experiences. In other words, CDZs.

13. Witnessing someone drink a glass of milk with a face contracting in an expression of disgust is presumed to be an example of the intuitive extreme of this continuum, the pre-reflective, empathetic level of representation. However, thinking about "what gift would please a foreign colleague" is an example of the more and reflective extreme, demanding logic, inference, cultural knowledge, and explicit knowledge about the inner life of others. These responses are explained as the product of ToM mechanisms by Keysers and Gazzola (2007: 194–195).

14. Although the critical debate surrounding the "posthuman" and "transhuman" is beyond the scope of this study, I recommend Clark's *Natural-Born Cyborgs: Minds, Technologies and the Future of Human Intelligence* (2003) and Ross's exploration of abused, dysfunctional, and (hyper)sexualized, as well as technologically augmented and even cloned bodies in *Primo Levi's Narratives of Embodiment: Containing the Human* (2011).

15. For the historical evolution of the concept and its part in late twentieth century debates see the long and detailed introduction to Kögler and Steuber 2000.

16. The presence, absence or degree of empathy has been measured through both embodied and discursive modes of analysis: through changes in heart rate and skin conductance (palm sweat), through studying perceptible (and imperceptible) facial reactions captured by electromyographic procedures (EMG), through Functional Magnetic Resonance Imaging (fMRI) and through questionnaires and surveys, asking subjects "how they feel or how they would act in certain situations, gathering responses through self-reports during or immediately after experiments and through surveys" (Keen 2006: 210).

17. [22] For more on ToM see Carruthers and Smith 1996 as well as Lisa Zunshine's *Why We Read Fiction: Theory of Mind and The Novel* in which she claims that this capacity underlies our understanding of fictional characters and, possibly, constitutes the main motivation for reading fiction at all.

18. This argument is pivotal to the discussion in Chapter 3 of this book.

19. This modularity is discussed in the next two chapters. Briefly, the theory arises from the recognition that so much information is

required to asses our immediate environment that we have evolved not only five senses but also a modular brain which processes different kinds of information via separate, expert brain regions. Thus our brains perform short-cuts that allow us to save time and move on, while gathering the maximum input we can process at a given time.

20. See Richardson and Spolsky 2004.

21. It is therefore also important to distinguish the Cognitive school from Literary Darwinism. See, for instance, Jonathan Kramnick (2011).

22. Different parts of the visual system have been shown to be involved depending on whether an object is represented for action or for perception (Decety et al. 1997: 1764). Similarly, distinct networks are activated when an action is designated for imitation, for imitation *and* reproduction, or for categorization and identification. Experiments show that recognition tasks are easier than imitation tasks, while semantic content is easily, almost automatically, related to meaningful actions (1767). More about the modularity and creativity of the visual system in Chapter 2.

23. Naturally, there exist great differences between playwrights such as Shakespeare, who left no stage directions at all, and writers such as Stoppard or Beckett for whom costume, stage tricks, lighting, music, volume etc. are stipulated in their directions and largely determine affect.

24. As explained above, this is a secondary process of conscious deliberation that takes place after the initial impact of physical response, but that is the nature of moral responsibility: active choice.

25. I use the term *relativism* to denote a long line of thinkers, most notably Nelson Goodman and Richard Rorty in our times, whose Relativist-Pragmatist positions deny the existence of a values system altogether, eschewing the possibility that there exists an independent reality beyond interpretation, believing in no vantage-point from which to gain purchase upon the conceptual scheme that determines reality. For an excellent volume of collected essays that debate the varieties, virtues, and vices of relativism see Krausz (1989). This issue is discussed in depth in Chapter 2.

1 "It Is Required You Do Awake Your Faith": Learning to Trust the Body through Performing *The Winter's Tale*

1. This chapter is a revised and modified version of the essay I contributed to the anthology *Performance and Cognition: Theatre Studies After the Cognitive Turn*, edited by Hart and McConachie (2006).

2. This understanding is not new. Richard Schechner describes two very different tribal ritual-cycles among the Australian Aborigines

and the Elema of New Guinea, both of which are "founded on the same belief in multiple, valid, equivalent, and reciprocating realities" (Schechner 1988: 49). However, the acceptance of multiplicity in Western Philosophical thinking is relatively recent.

3. Heidegger, of course, ardently resisted closed dualities and criticized Plato's use of binaries in *Being and Time*.

4. Cavell attributes the coining of this phrase to Winnicott in his discussion of "the good enough mother."

5. Cavell compares Leontes's laments that knowledge is like a poisonous spider (II.i.40–45) with the philosopher David Hume's sense of being "cursed, or sickened, in knowing more than his fellows about the fact of knowing itself" (Cavell 1987:197), which Hume calls the "malady" of knowledge. I deliberately use the term *reason*, because it is precisely the mistake of limiting "knowledge" to logic that breeds the malady.

6. Robert Green, *Pandosto, or The Triumph of Time* (1588). King Pandosto's wife Bellaria, "to show how she liked him whom her husband loved," (159) attends to and entertains Egistus King of Sicilia with such "familiar courtesy" that she could perhaps be suspected. For instance, she "oftentimes came herself into his bed-chamber to see that nothing should be amiss" (159). This is not given as justification of Pandosto's "flaming jealousy" (160). However, Bellaria and Egistus are described as "silly souls" (160) who, though innocently, may have lacked a certain measure of tact or propriety, spending too much time in one another's company, allowing Pandosto's "disordinate fancy" to "misconstrue of their too private familiarity" (160).

7. King Leontes (Everyman), by rejecting Grace (Hermione), killing Childhood (Mamillus), and banishing natural Innocence (Perdita), is left bereft, lonely, and on the verge of despair. He is, however, taught humility through suffering but is not finally denied Heaven's grace. See Milward (1964).

8. Unless one argues that she was dead for sixteen years etc.

9. Robert W. Corrigen has argued that this hybrid genre is endemic to times of unrest (Corrigen 1979: 222), but it may be argued that almost every period in history has included elements of unrest. Indeed, Stephen Greenblatt (1973: 348) argues that, as an artist, Sidney was not concerned with re-establishing the stability that his times seem to have lost but, rather, to be a "connoisseur of doubt" (351).

10. Cavell also detects a competition between Leontes and his son over who has the right to tell this tale and suggests that the play unfolds a reversed oedipal conflict: not one in which the son wishes to replace the father, but one generated by "the father's wish to replace or remove his son" (Cavell 1987: 199). In his mad state, Leontes wants there to be no counting or recounting; in other words, he wants

there to be nothing. And that is what he achieves: his son dies, his daughter is lost. This is, of course, far from traditional interpretations of the death of the son, for which see Hunter (186–203). On the connection with the ongoing conflict between King James and his son Henry, see Palmer (331). As for Perdita being "lost," Frances E. Dolan argues that *The Winter's Tale* is most "like an old tale" (V.iii.117) because it replicates an all too familiar story of infant abandonment. She insists that we not efface the fact that Perdita was never "lost" but was cast out by her violent father. By dwelling on the language of loss, argues Dolan, "the play prepares for forgiveness by sparing Leontes the direct, criminalized agency...helping us to repress our knowledge of his crucial role in "losing" his children." (Dolan 1994: 167).

11. III.iii.90–100 Antigonus is reported by the clown to have been eaten by a bear. It is a matter of directorial choice whether or not the audience sees or merely hears of this event. In the 2003 RSC production, a huge bear devoured him on stage.

12. Polixenes commands Camillo: "If you know ought which does behove my Knowledge / Thereof to be inform'd, imprison't not / In ignorant concealment" (I.ii.395–7). Yet both Leontes and Polixenes are weakened by inform'd knowledge and restored by concealment. Camillo, Florizel, Perdita, Autolycus, Paulina, and Hermione each in turn conceal knowledge, thereby correcting the faults of others (Palmer 1995: 335). The issue of Hermione's "resurrection" is discussed at length below.

13. Alternative political contexts to the religio-political theme are offered by Donna B. Hamilton's reading (1993), which reminds us that the play was written just as King James's proposal to unify England with Scotland was hotly debated, convincingly arguing that Shakespeare deploys the literary trend of using a pastoral setting for political commentary and replicates the particular rhetoric of the Union controversy in *The Winter's Tale*. Kaplan and Eggert (1994) suggest a reading of the play as an allegory of Anne Boleyn's downfall and Elizabeth's bastardization. Landau (2003) claims it also resonate with Henry VIII's initial rejection of Katherine of Aragon. And Daryl W. Palmer explores the connections between this winter's tale and that of Richard Chancellor who "discovered Russia" in 1553. The ensuing diplomatic ties with the Muscovites were apparently accompanied by proliferating tales of strange customs, jealousies, and violent deeds that fueled the English imagination, and it is by no chance, argues Palmer, that Shakespeare mentions Hermione's father is "The Emperor of Russia" (III.ii.119). In Shakespeare's source, it is not Pandosto's wife Balleria, but Egistus's wife, who is the daughter of the Russian emperor (*Pandosto* 164), thus providing Egistus with powerful alliances that dissuade Pandosto from waging war upon Sicilia. The fact that Pandosto cannot effectively reap

his revenge upon Egistus is given as the prime reason for his turning all his anger towards Balleria (*Pandosto* 164).

14. Carol Chillington Rutter argues that in almost every Shakespeare play, men are given more lines, while women express themselves through *actions*. Women's centrality to their respective plays is revealed, therefore, in *performance*. Thus, attending to the body means attending to "theatre's 'feminine' unruliness and the unpredictable, not to say promiscuous, theory-resisting effects performance generates" (Rutter 2001: xv).

15. See also Decety J. et al. (1997); Grèzes et al. (1998); Iacoboni et al. (1999).

16. Clinical evidence of a similar phenomenon is also found in so-called "imitation-behavior" (Lhermitte 1986), according to which humans observing another agent in action "generate a plan to do the same action, or an image of doing it, themselves"—whether or not this is translated into actual motor movements.

17. One must keep in mind that the entire Christian religion rests on belief in Christ's incarnation and resurrection. Everyone in Shakespeare's audience (bar perhaps a few individuals) believed in *that* miracle.

2 "A Doubling of Immortality:" Cognitive Inter(con)textuality and Tom Stoppard's *Travesties*

1. Thus Spoke Zarathustra was written in four parts between 1883 and 1885. At first it was only published privately. The first public edition was published in 1891.

2. I use the term *relativism* to denote a long line of thinkers, most notably Nelson Goodman and Richard Rorty in our times, whose Relativist-Pragmatist positions deny the existence of a values system altogether, eschewing the possibility that there exists an independent reality beyond interpretation, believing in no vantage-point form which to gain purchase upon the conceptual scheme that determines reality. For an excellent volume of collected essays that debate the varieties, virtues, and vices of relativism see Krausz (1989).

3. Once eighteenth century interest in the orient, and in distant and yet equally sophisticated cultures (China, India, Turkey) took root, a new kind of relativism was born. This awareness of cultural and historical time-place specifics, and of values as context-bound, did not, however, disturb the self-righteous confidence of most Westerners in their superiority. In the nineteenth-century confusion overtook certainty. The effects of the French Revolution (its dream and its demise) upon both social idealism and political theory, the accumulating (and accelerating) effects of industrialism, with its attendant social upheavals and injustices, were matched with gradual social reforms

that paved the way to the establishment of a democratic parliamentary rule; Wesleyan Methodist revival and its Puritan ethics; Darwinism, which shook the foundations of both science and religion; the rise of Utilitarian philosophy, which unsettled the previous criterion for value judgment. Almost every notion proposed in this period has a directly antithetical contemporary opposite with which to contend, creating an environment of such dizzyingly swift and unpredictable changes, and dialectic thought patterns, that a strain of radical skepticism became almost inevitable. But while Walter Pater famously retuned to a Humean skepticism, Mathew Arnold advocated an opposing view. Although aware of the "baneful notion that there is no such thing as a high, correct standard in intellectual matters; that every one may as well take his own way" ("The Literary Influence of Academies." *Essays in Criticism* 66; Houghton 33), Arnold held that the anarchy of individualism can and should be effectively contained by the authority of Culture, a force able to fix "standards that are real!" *(Culture and Anarchy* 1 51; Houghton 33).

4. *The Will To Power* was published posthumously in 1901. This fragment, however, is dated 1887.

5. Many of Nietzsche's ideas are pertinent to the main arguments made in this book, although his political theories remain highly controversial, particularly his belief in the necessity of a three-tiered society. His view that "inequality of rights is the only condition of there being rights at all. [. . .] A high civilization is a pyramid: it can stand only upon a broad base" (1889: 220) stands in direct opposition to the Sentimentalist-democratic ideals discussed in Chapter 3 of this book.

6. Talmon argues that if defining the ideal constitutes limitless possibilities, and so searching for it requires only openness but no fixed goal, the project becomes self-defeating. The result is what Schlegel identified as *Sehensucht*—a never appeased longing. On the one hand a strident, solipsistic, individual quest, on the other hand a longing for total immersion in an all-embracing oneness. See Talmon pp.135–162.

7. Wilde's *The Picture of Dorian Gray* had already, in 1890, explored the dangers inherent in a purely aesthetic view of life. The wittiness of Lord Henry may be charming at the dinner table, but if his ethos of indifference is put into practice, its subordination of morality to beauty becomes fatal.

8. His political analysis rests on the view that because postmodern thought had reduced "all truth-claims to a species of rhetorical imposition," critique and principled opposition were disarmed. The masses, argues Norris, were persuaded that majority consensus triumphed. If the U.S. president managed to persuade enough people of his version of the truth—that became truth. Thus, not a skepticism,

but a terrifying "Uncritical Theory" invaded international relations, particularly those controlled by the western superpowers. For "elections were no longer won or lost on the strength of valid arguments, appeals to moral justice, or even to enlightened self-interest on the part of a reasonably well-informed electorate. What counted now was the ability to seize the high ground of PR and public opinion management by adopting strategies that faithfully mirrored the perceived selfimage of the times" (Norris 3).

9. To my very great regret, due to the strict permission and distribution limitations of Grove Atlantic Press, I have had to cut almost all citations from the play. Discussion of Stoppard's word-games and humor in this chapter is thus greatly hampered.

10. In a review from 1977, Stoppard "scoffs at the idea that facts are context-bound and theory laden," calling relativism not only "false" but "silly. Daft. Not very bright . . . wicked" (Mackenzie 575). This statement not only counters Rorty and Kuhn, but also Fish (1980). However, Rorty famously argues that we should converse, not because Socratic dialogue is a means to an end (truth, value, virtue) but an end in itself: conversation should replace the concept of reason (1982: 166–8).

11. Being so very chaotic, Stoppard's plays have invited description in terms of Chaos Theory. Indeed, his play *Arcadia* explicitly concerns this theory. Appropriation of the scientific theory of Chaos has found enthusiastic advocates in the humanities, chief among them Katherine Hayles, who infers that the new "paradigm of orderly disorder" represented by chaos theory signifies a conceptual revolution in modern culture as a whole (1990 and 1991). She has attempted to establish parallels between chaos theory and various poststructuralist philosophical positions, including those of Derrida and Foucault. However, Carl Matheson and Evan Kirchoff (1997) show convincingly that chaos does not have the power to change the very paradigm conception of space-time in the way relativity or quantum science did. It challenges a long-accepted link between determinism and predictability but, essentially, "it adds to what has gone before rather than overturning it," being co-opted by, rather than transforming, multiple fields of inquiry (Matheson and Kirchoff 31). Instead, not only do they show that chaos and deconstruction are not isomorphic in any interesting sense, and that there is no evidence of a substantial causal connection between them, but they argue that "Chaos is loosely analogous to, if anything, classical philosophical skepticism. It is a scientific reformulation of the Lockean worry that, although our scrutable world of sense is determined by the external world, we may never come to know about that external world. Alternatively, one could detect shades of Kant in chaos theory, whereby the noumenal is necessary for the phenomenal, although the noumenal

remains forever outside our ken. As such, it is not postmodernist or poststructuralist; [. . .] it is an instantiation of the problem which gave rise to philosophical modernism: nature as necessary and determinate, yet unknowable" (Matheson and Kirchoff 37). To this must be added Stoppard's own testimony that he has "no interest in anarchic or unstructured art" (Stoppard to Eichelbaum 1997: 105).

12. Dada was a movement committed to showing disgust for the senseless values of the society that invented trench-warfare. Social decadence and political mayhem were perceived to have done away with logic, rendering nonsense and "completely pointless" activities (Tzara in *Travesties* 27) the only appropriate response. Dada "art" was intended to shock, creating the greatest possible degree of misunderstanding between the performer/artist and audience. Surrealism may be said to be a development that refined Dada's call for desecrating the rational into an exploration through the arts of the mysteries of the irrational mind—a form of Romanticism repeating itself with a difference.

13. Opening of Act II. Carr is at this stage disguised as Tristan, the decadent nihilist younger brother of Jack, the library-persona of the real Tristan (*Travesties* 46–53).

14. Henry Carr, the narrator of *Travesties*, played the part of Algernon ("not Ernest, the other one") in Joyce's 1918 production. In his daydreaming at present he confuses himself with the characters of both Algernon and Ernest, and rages against Joyce who underpaid him for his performance, and then surpassed him in fame and glory by becoming a revered writer. Tristan Tzara (1896–1963), the Dada artist, who ought to be better suited to play the zany Algernon character, is instead assigned the part of the earnest John Worthing (Jack-Ernest). The two men do, however, fall in love with the women Wilde writes for them, Carr-Algernon marrying Cecily, and Tzara-Ernest marrying Gwendolyn. Gwendolyn, Carr's younger sister in *Travesties*, and Algernon's cousin in *The Importance of Being Earnest*, is closer in character to Wilde's Cecily, who falls for the unconventional Algernon. Cecily, Lenin's devotee, with whom Carr falls in love, as Algernon does in *Earnest*, is closer in character to Wilde's Gwendolyn, who falls in love with the earnest *The Importance of Being Earnest*. So that Stoppard may be said to have reversed the female characters as well as the male ones to "correct" Joyce's miscasting. To add to this confusion, Bennet, Carr's manservant in *Travesties*, is named after the historical English Consul in Zurich in 1917, for whom the historical Carr worked in reality. He is almost a one-to-one reproduction of Wilde's Lane. (Bennet is Carr's superior in their unflattering appearance in *Ulysses*). Meantime James Joyce (1882–1941) is not only as officious as Lady Bracknell, but the comparison between them is made explicit in the scene in which

Joyce interrogates Tzara, just as Lady Bracknell interrogates Jack-Ernest in *The Importance of Being Earnest*. He does so, however, in a style reminiscent of the constabulary style of the "Ithaca" section in *Ulysses*. Lady Bracknell is also echoed by Lenin when he talks of the failed 1905 revolution, "to lose one revolution is unfortunate. To lose two would look like carelessness!" (T 58). Indeed, Vladimir Lenin (1870–1924) and his wife Nadezda (Nadya) Krupskaya, are at once presented as earnest revolutionaries and farcical book-worms, scheming to disguise themselves in order to re-enter Russia but ending up resembling Chasubel and Miss Prism. Travesty indeed.

15. When I read Yeats's wonderful play *The Only Jealousy of Emer* I cried. When I went to see it performed (National Arts Club, New York, directed by Sam McCready, April 2006)—aware that the production had followed, with remarkable fidelity, the directions of the playwright—I felt almost no emotion at all. The symbolist stage, intriguing and challenging as it may be, entirely cancels out the powerful emotional impact of the text. Once again, this was part of Yeats's design but, in my view, counterproductive.

16. This may be a wink at Hume's famous ridiculing of "the monkish virtues" of ascetic self-denial in *An Inquiry Concerning the Principles of Morals* (1751).

17. Like *Travesties*, *The Real Thing* concerns art and politics, but it is most of all, like *The Winter's Tale*, about love, jealousy, and (in)fidelity. In both plays, the central theme is the difficulty of discerning what is "real." *Jumpers*—Stoppard's professedly theist play—gives voice to relativism, utilitarianism, and logical positivism, but sides uncompromisingly with the liberal believer George. *Arcadia*, considers chaos theory. Both Thomasina and Valentina believe mathematics can discover unalterable truths, but find that even equations cannot guarantee stable patterns. At the same time, *Arcadia* also suggests that when structure and stability emerge they should be acknowledged.

18. One of Stoppard's identifying structural characteristics is beginning his plays with a false front—a scene the audience thinks "real" and discovers is not. In accordance, this opening scene in the library turns out to be entirely imagined by old Carr.

19. This is why "iterability" is so central to (post)Derridian theory. The principle of iterability holds that in order to be understood, the utterance has to be recognizable. The principle of citationality holds that because language *is* iterable, it has a tendency to carry associations from one context to another. As Derrida explained: "Every sign, linguistic or non-linguistic, spoken or written . . . can be *cited*, put between quotation marks; in so doing it can break with any given context, engendering an infinity of new contexts in a manner which is absolutely illimitable. This does not imply that the mark is valid outside of

a context, but on the contrary, that there are only contexts without any center or absolute anchoring [*ancrage*]" (Derrida 1977: 185).

20. Margaret Gold (1978) refers to George Bernard Shaw as "the second of the Dadas in *Travesties*," comparing Carr and Tzara's exchange to that of Don Juan and Mephistopheles in *Man and Superman* (Gold 61). She also compares Bennet (the well informed butler) to Shaw's chauffeur mechanic 'enry Straker, while viewing Tzara as a travesty of Shaw himself—artist and socialist—who loses the art battle to Joyce and the political battle to Lenin (1978: 62). *Travesties*, she continues, picks up where *Heartbreak House* left off. Shaw complained of the bourgeois complacent culture of superficial leisure, which failed to understand the enormity of either the First World War or the Russian Revolution until it was too late. Indeed the same can be said of Carr in *Travesties*. But Stoppard "carries the whole problem a step closer to the abyss that yawns between ordinary men and Supermen. Men like Joyce and Lenin who are children of Genius and Destiny elude the chains of common reasoning" . . . (65).

21. What's more, as Paul Grice (1975) argues, communication is a form of inter-personal social contract which relies on the "Co-operative Principl" and "implicature."

22. Recall Horace's *Ars Poetica*, in which he directs the poet how to captivate the audience, teach, please and move them, and thereby win immortality.

23. When a ball is kicked, humans easily identify the kicker as the cause of motion. But when an object seems to move of its own volition we automatically interpret the cause of motion as (necessarily invisible) intention. "The contrast between visible and invisible is, of course, a fundamental, profoundly human distinction . . . engendered by a mind or brain that is utterly committed to explanation but capable of realizing the commitment with no other tool than that of cause" (Premack 1995: 207, my italics).

24. I am using "text" in the broadest sense of the word, including not only written texts, but any codified form of human discourse, from (unconscious) cultural norms to complex literary texts.

25. Any sophisticated text has multiple layers of meaning, and it is clear that only few in Stoppard's audience are able to pick up even a fraction of the dizzyingly varied sources which he (mis)quotes and parodies. But at the same time, his play cannot allow its entire force to lie in such (often obscure) references. In order to communicate with its audience, the play's general gist must be self-explanatory. And so it is.

26. Hutcheon worries that the necessity for shared codes of reference in parody creates "potential for elitism." In my view, though culturally-specific knowledge is indispensable to parody, it needn't be elitist. Derrida observed that *no speech-event* may signify unless it repeats a "code [. . .] conforming with an iterable model . . . identifiable as

a citation" (Derrida 1977: 192). Indeed, it is essential to be familiar with American slang in order to understand rap music, yet that is hardly elitist.

27. This claim stands in contrast to Margaret Rose's argument in *Parody/Metafiction* (1979) that parody in literary history creates discontinuity by rejecting previous works.

28. *The Republic* Book X. Since Plato's "theory of forms" determined that art is merely an imitation of the Phenomenal dimension of existence, which is itself merely a shadow of the Ideal realm of absolute abstraction. According to this view, art is twice removed from perfection and therefore completely useless. (He mistakenly calculates it as being three-times removed). Plato held that only dialectic philosophy can attempt to describe the Ideal. Aristotle countered this argument, but it is of interest to note that Oscar Wilde insisted that art in fact imitates the Ideal directly, occupying a dimension above the Phenomenal. Moreover, he asserted that "all art is quite useless" (1890:6), and this is its greatest merit, since the function of art is anti-utilitarian.

29. In fact, Stoppard originally thought of calling the play *Prism*, another image of refraction and multiplicity (*The Times*, June 8, 1974: 9).

30. The historical Tzara even changed his name from Samuel Rosenstock to one that better exemplified his call for self-definition. Tzara means "motherland" in Romanian.

31. Stoppard once said that his plays are "a lot to do with the fact that I just don't know . . . One thing I feel sure about is that a materialistic view of history is an insult to the human race" (Stoppard to Hudson et al. Delaney 65–6).

32. Because he acknowledges that interviewers invite him to reflect, retroactively, on a playwriting process that may have been a combination of research, chance, epiphany, and whim, Stoppard has suggested that his interviews should be printed with "a warning, like on cigarette packets. A warning which states: this profile is in the middle truth range. Don't inhale" (Stoppard to Bradshaw 1977: 90). All citations from interviews in this chapter are therefore to be considered "middle truths."

33. Apart from being one of any magician's elementary tricks, the rabbit also reminds us of *Alice in Wonderland* which features so prominently as one of the intertexts of the play.

34. Joyce's agreement to rewrite some of Wilde's play in order to accommodate Carr's fashion obsession, for the sake of getting two pounds, is not only suspiciously lacking in artistic integrity but also demeaningly money-oriented. It smacks of the greed of capitalism, which Tzara gives as the cause for the war (*Travesties* 22); though in Joyce's case capitalist ethics are practiced for the sake of the art-war.

35. This echoes the theory of the Romantic-Modernist hagiography of the artist. See Julia Reinhard (1996).

36. Mathew Arnold argued that "in truth, the word 'God' is used in most cases as by no means a term of science or exact knowledge, but a term of poetry and eloquence;" God is actually "a literary term" (*Literature and Dogma* 1873). By extension, he argued, all poetry reveals a quasi-religious function. The Modernists took this a step further, considering the artist to be analogous to a prophet-priest. Modernist literature, moreover, often endorses a strictly hierarchical social order, whether harking back to ancient chivalric codes of honor and a feudal society clearly divided into three estates (Yeats), or in advocating a Nietzschean tripartite system for consciousness and the need for a social-pyramid (Eliot, Lewis). The Modernists adopted these ideas partly as a means of containing the vulgar, popular and ultimately (to their minds) destructive elements of society—which include both the bourgeoisie that Lenin hated and the proletariat he idealized.

37. Heuvel describes Stoppard's work as "humanized postmodernism (or postmodernized humanism)" as he has "essentially made his career as playwright by having it both ways" (Heuvel 219). *Travesties* incorporates contesting cultural narratives but "reduces these conflicts to pure spectacle, unhinged from actual historical referents and devoid of modernist anxiety and overt critical stance towards such mutually antagonistic viewpoints" (Heuvel 220). He also argues that by refusing to determine one view as right, the play "produces a sense of what Jameson calls "hyperspace," a disorienting but not necessarily debilitating map of ideas existing without a center of gravity or absolute cartographical code" (Heuvel 220). I disagree on both accounts. I think Stoppard's text makes it very clear which narrative is "right" in his view, and this is crucial.

38. To understand the meaning of a descriptive expression, it is not enough to recognize it or even be able to use it, one must be able to "call to mind the ideas, both linguistic and empirical, embodied in the mental schemas and commonly held to be associated with the referent in the given language community" (Arbib and Hesse 154); or as Wittgenstein termed it, to "grasp" the "concept." In other words, pre-existing neuronal assemblies or semantic clusters associated with a particular concept already lodged in our long-term memory—the CDZs explained in the introduction tot his book. These can then be modified, altered, annexed.

39. In an interview in 1968 Stoppard said that "I feel some guilt about being a writer. Probably all artists feel guilty . . . Artists are made to feel decorators, embroiderers . . . " Kelly calls *Travesties* a partial "exorcism" of this guilt ("Something to Declare." *The Sunday Times* 25 February 1968 47; cited by Kelly (1990): 382).

40. Self-creation, the creation of a personal narrative and the possibility of re-writing that narrative are the themes developed in Chapter 3, in which I discuss Timberlake Wertenbaker's *Our Country's Good*.

41. Lane's book, in which he supposedly documents the accounts of the household, turns out to be a cover for his plundering of the Moncrieff wine cellar. Cecily's love-letters and her diary give completely fictional accounts of her relationship with the equally fictional Ernest. Cecily further confuses life with art when she explains that as "a very young girl's record of her own thoughts and impressions," her diary is "consequently meant for publication" (*Earnest* II 341). The conflict between Cecily and Gwendolyn over Earnest is in fact conducted by reference to texts—"Our little country newspaper, The *Morning Post*" and both their diaries (*Earnest* II 345–6). Gwendolyn's diary may well be as fictional as Cecily's (or the newspapers they read), as its greatest function is to have "something sensational to read on the train" (*Earnest* II 346). Lady Bracknell carries her list of eligible young men, and Jack himself has recourse to the Army Lists to prove his identity. All the documents of "Miss Cardew's birth, baptism, whooping-cough, registration, vaccination, confirmation and the measles; both the German and the English variety" are also in tact in the Court Guides in Jack's keeping (*Earnest* III 356).

42. Carr refers to Joyce's text in words that echo Lady Bracknell's reference to Miss Prism's "three-volume novel of more than usually revolting sentimentality" (*Earnest* III 360): "inordinate in length and erratic in style" (*Travesties* 70). The fact that it is "remotely connected to midwifery" (*Travesties* 70) makes it all the more apt.

43. Scientists call this "motocentric" rather than "visuocentric." See Clark (1998) and also Heidegger (1927).

44. 2–17 May 2003 and directed by Richard Baron.

45. For discussion of the ritual significance of symbolic monuments and spaces, such as Capitol Hill, Tiananmen Square, or the Berlin Wall as sites for the staging of improvised/revolutionary demonstrations, which are fundamentally theatrical, see Schechner (1992).

46. in an interview with Michael Billington, 1975.

47. *Prudent skepticism*, of the kind that encourages doubt—in the form of intelligent questioning that counterweighs blind faith, dogmatism and tyranny—is both intellectually sound and wise. However, surrendering to *unqualified skepticism*, which in its extremity leads to nihilism and pessimism is, I argue, self-destructive.

48. Lyotard's notion of the "unpresentable" is borrowed from Kant's logic of the sublime, which takes place when "the imagination fails to present an object which might, if only in principle, come to match a concept" (Lyotard 147). However, Claire Colebrook (2000) reminds us that while Kant acknowledged that no pre-representational world in itself could be *known*, he nevertheless maintained that it was necessary to assume its existence. If knowledge is representation then it must be a representation *of* something (Colebrook 53). Both the pessimistic view of representation that longs to return to a world

that is lived as present, and the utopian view that imagines a point beyond representation, a "radical homelessness" (Colebrook 48) that expresses a desire to overcome all commitments to presence in the celebration of a differential, non-autonomous, and post-human writing, are shown by Colebrook to express nostalgia (Colebrook 59).

3   From Empathy to Sympathy: Staging Change and Conciliation in Timberlake Wertenbaker's *Our Country's Good*

1. The division of *The Theory of Moral Sentiments* into parts is irregular. Thus, Parts I and II are referenced here as Part, Section, Chapter, Paragraph (such as Part I I.i.1) but, as I read an online version of the book, there are no page references. Further, not all parts have section divisions (as in Part II and IV), or they have sections but no chapters (as in Part VI). I try to make this explicit in the references.

2. First performed at the Royal Court Theatre in London in 1988, it was awarded the Laurence Olivier/BBC Award for Best New Play and the New York Drama Critics' Circle Award for Best New Foreign Play. The play also won Wertenbaker the Evening Standard Award for Most Promising Playwright, 1988.

3. Sentimentalism in England may be traced back to the Cambridge Platonists, but is usually attributed to Anthony Ashley-Cooper, the 3rd Earl of Shaftesbury (1671–1713) in his attack on Locke in *Characteristics of Men, Manners, Opinions, Times* (1711). Shaftesbury held that Lock's account of the senses does not accommodate that "inward eye" which, through inborn sentiments of pity, benevolence, love and gratitude, shapes and determine moral values and judgments. In turn, Shaftesbury influenced Francis Hutcheson (1694–1746), David Hume (1711–1776) and Adam Smith (1723–1790).

4. *The Theory of Moral Sentiments* was published in 1759 during his tenure of the Chair of Moral Philosophy at the University of Glasgow. Six authorized editions of *TMS* were published in Smith's lifetime. Edition 2 appeared in 1761. Editions 3 (1767), 4 (1774), and 5 (1781) of *TMS* differ little from Edition 2. Edition 6, however, published shortly before Smith's death in 1790, contains very extensive additions and other significant changes. Thus, the historical Arthur Phillip could not have read this final version before setting off to New South Wales in 1789. However, he may well have read one of the earlier versions; his policies certainly suggest that he did.

5. After 1794 honor, duty, and rightness replaced sentiment, which was relegated to the private sphere of male-female relations and was most particularly associated with women and fiction. The Romantic notion of sentiment was already inextricably bound to self interest. (There is good reason why, in his *Biographia Literaria*, Coleridge articulated

his initial attraction to Wordsworth's "genius"—so famously characterized by the "a spontaneous overflow of powerful feelings"—by explaining that he detected in his poetry "manly reflection and human associations" (IV: 79). But sentiment was irrevocably established as necessary in intersubjective relationships.

6. The historical Captain Tench recorded that many convicts were incapable of articulating themselves in Standard English. It is likely therefore that the historical convict-players who were permitted to perform a play were better spoken than the majority of their fellows. Accordingly, all Keneally's players are perfectly able to articulate themselves in Standard English from the start.

7. Weeks' argument is more relevant to Wertenbaker's play *Case to Answer* (1980), in which Sylvia comes to despise the cultural oppression of her husband and his jargon-ridden, Marxist sociology which, by "continually ignoring" her language, makes her "feel inadequate." She accuses Niko of "theft of language:" "By making me doubt its value, you took it away from me…Having frozen my language you substituted yours, thereby transmitting your values, beliefs, convictions and thoughts." Weeks' claims are also relevant to *The Grace of Mary Traverse* (1985) in which Mary's discovery that language can be used to disguise rather than reveal meaning initially produces, as in the case of Leontes in *The Winter's Tale*, a sense of nausea: "I feel a cripple's anger. I can't touch or smell the world" (13). She explains, "It's my father who taught me to talk, sir. He didn't suspect he'd also be teaching me to think" (38). But this is precisely what Governor Phillip is aiming for—to teach the convicts to think for themselves. Thus mistaking Phillip for Niko or Giles is unjustified. For Liz, language creates opportunity where once there was despair.

8. It is not necessary for the purposes of this study to enter into British politics at the time, beyond the recognition that, like the trends in postmodern theory addressed in Chapter 2, great emphasis was placed upon sectarian divisions. In retrospect, it is possible to see that in 1988 Thatcher's power and influence were already waning, but most Britains at the time were still embroiled in the effects of the volatile disagreements of preceding years The class divisions, which persist in English culture to a far greater extent than in other European counties, may create a sense of insurmountable difference, but they never predetermined political affinities: there are aristocratic liberals and working class conservatives. However, in the 1980s, in addition to the cumulative effects of an economic recession, unemployment, and massive immigration from the ex-colonies, there existed radical and often violent animosity between those who supported or objected to the war in The Falklands, and between the National Front white-supremacist 'skinheads' and the pluralistic, post-punk, 2Tone 'ska' culture. This was a period of polarizing oppositions; everything from

governmental policies to pop-culture seemed inflected by mutually exclusive binaries, and by the politics of domination and power-games at that. See, as a start, Adonis, Andrew and Tim Hames eds. *A Conservative Revolution? The Tatcher-Reagan Decade in Perspective.* Manchester: Manchester UP, 1994. And Reynolds, Simon. *Rip It Up and StartAagain :Post-Punk 1978–84.* London: Faber and Faber, 2005.

 9. This is, of course, an ongoing debate in political ethics. There are those who argue that Socialism, and even more so Communism, purport to benefit the people, while actually relying on their continual subjugation (for instance, Sullivan 152). Whether or not this is the case, Wertenbaker suggest that republican ideas need not be rejected just because the French revolutionaries abused them. Neither should modern-day versions of the government of the people be overshadowed by the brutality of Soviet Communism. Wertenbaker's message seems to be that supplementing contractual social theory with Sentimentalism—with benevolence—may possibly make way for humanitarian rule. Indeed Smith's model of conduct was aimed at creating a "decent" society. At the height of Thatcher's power, when Wertenbaker's play was first performed, both conservatives and liberals were more often concerned with the rights of individuals and groups than with establishing agreement regarding what a "decent" society may imply. Still today, as I argued in the previous chapter, the Postmodern endorsement of pluralism in all its forms seems to forestall any consensus, let alone a shared code of conduct or values. And yet, few liberals in the West are likely to reject Smith's basic assumption that all civilizations depend upon the fostering and regulation of respect for life and property, concern for the common good, and moral accountability. These concerns are as pertinent to today's world, governed by global capitalism, as they were in the early eighteenth century. That is, in great measure, why Wertenbaker's play can tie the 1790s to the late 1980s with such seamlessness, and why her play still resonates with audiences in 2011.

10. It appears that the first female convict to be executed was a woman by the name of Ann Davis alias Judith Jones, executed October 1789 for breaking into Robert Sideway's house and stealing articles and clothes (Collins 1975: 6).

11. *Involuntary Emotional Identification* implies an "involuntary suffusion of feeling which is manifested in a physical way, no matter how slight, and triggered by a perceived or imagined sign of feeling, or a perceived or imagined condition which implies feeling, in a living creature or creatures" (Levy 1997: 181). *Sympathetic Projection* denotes "the faculty or capacity for imagining the unarticulated, even unobserved, feeling and/or motives of another living creature, or of attributing feelings and/or motives to an inanimate objects in nature

or art" which is closest to the original meaning of Einfulung, borrowed from the German." It is an act of imagination which can be either willed or unwilled. *Sympathetic Understanding*, Levy defines as "the faculty or capacity for being attuned, at an emotional level, to the unarticulated feelings and/or motives of another living creature and, in particular, being attuned to signals of disturbance or distress. This is what a successful spouse, lover, parent or pet owner does. It is what a good Method actor does. It is also what a skillful and practiced therapist does" (182).

12. Midshipman Harry Brewer embodies a kind of middleman between the officer class and the convicts. When Harry admits, "The officers may look down on me now, but what if they found out that I used to be an embezzler?" Clark is unresponsive: "Harry you should keep these things to yourself" (*Country* 7). Harry's good nature nonetheless provides a bridge between the two classes, though this is developed in the novel to a far greater extent than in the play.

13. Basic emotions have long been identified as a universal human feature (also shared, to an extent, by other mammals). See Darwin 1872 and Ekman 1983 and 1992. .

14. In the novel, on first considering Mary for the play, he is "seduced" by the image of her reading aloud to the convict women aboard *Lady Penrhyn*. Her literacy, childish innocence, and motherly kindness are fused in this image; words and deeds merge.

15. The historical Ralph's journal, *The Journal and Letters of Lt. Ralph Clark 1787–1792*, indicates genuine and powerful love for his wife and child, "the best Woman and Sweetest of Boys" (Clark 13). It also describes overwhelming misery at having to leave them as well as recurring sea-sickness and dreams/nightmares fed by love and fear for them and the habit of ritually kissing Betsy's picture and a lock of the boy's hair (Clark 20) on Sundays. The journal also indicates an arrogant intolerance towards the female convicts aboard the *Friendship*—"dammed whores...abandoned wretches" (Clark 12). There is a running theme of dreams, nightmares, and Aboriginal lore running through the novel. This is given some attention in the play but I shall not be discussing that here. It may nonetheless be interesting to note that Richard Schechner connects the Greek word *drama*—to do, to act—with the old English word for dream—*dram*, and to the Aborigines' view of the dream-state as one in which we share in the creativity of nature. "The creative condition is identical with trances, dances ecstasies; in short shamanism" (Schechner 1988: 41–43).

16. It is intriguing to note that the historical Ralph's journal records events between March 9, 1787 and March 10, 1788. Then there is a gap, and it is only resumed on February 15, 1790. Thus the whole period of playmaking is nonexistent, and the romance with Mary

unrecorded. However, other records indicate that he did cohabit with her and that she bore him a daughter, christened Alicia after his wife, on December 16, 1791. This event also falls in a conspicuous gap of nearly seven weeks in the resumed journal. There is no way of verifying the possibility that a whole volume of the journal was deliberately destroyed, but this seems very likely. The historic Ralph did not, however, direct the convict-play. In the novel, he sees himself as the grand playmaker, the theater manager, and takes delight in that creativity without taking part in the performance. Second, he senses that the convicts "wanted the play all lag, all convict," that they relished a sense of "exclusiveness" (Keneally 71). From the start he expects a "tribal magic" (Keneally 72) to envelop the participants and from the first rehearsal he is witness to the "expansion" of the convicts' presences. In Wertenbaker's play he is an active participant in the production and the performance.

17. As mentioned in note 8, there can be little doubt that Wertenbaker is also creating an analogy with England in 1988, tying her claims to the political climate of the time and the liberal dream of better social cohesion. If this were a Stoppard play, there would probably be a song by The Specials playing in the background of this scene.

18. Criticism of over-strict reasoning, privileging rank and money while practicing indifference to the suffering of others, exploitation of them and brutality towards them are of course also expressed in the literature of the time: Defoe, Richardson, Fielding, Wollstonecraft, and others.

19. Basic emotions have long been identified as a universal human feature (also shared, to an extent, by other mammals). These include: fear, happiness, surprise, sadness, anger and disgust (Darwin 1872; Ekman 1983, 1992).

20. I explore this claim - and its potential for negative effect - at length in "Too far gone in disgust": Mirror Neurons and the Manipulation of Embodied Responses in The Libertine." Configurations 16:3 (2010): 400–426.

21. The Natyasastra, compiled in India between the second century BCE and the second century CE, describes in great detail various facial and bodily poses and expressions needed to perform the "eight basic emotions" of classical Indian dance theatre: love, happiness, sadness (or grief), anger, energy, fear, disgust, and surprise. "A ninth emotion, peace or sublime tranquility (*shanta*) was added later" (Schechner 266). Schechner thus challenges the acting technique made famous by Konstantine Stanislavski, by which actors recall past emotional experiences ("affective memory") in order to re-create an emotion on stage.

22. Though only a small collection of subcortical sites induce emotion, these sites nonetheless process different emotions to varying degrees.

"For instance, sadness consistently activates the ventromedial prefrontal cortex, hypothalamus, and brain stem, while anger or fear activate neither the prefrontal cortex nor hypothalamus. Brainstem activation is shared by all three, but intense hypothalamic and ventromedial prefrontal activation appears specific to sadness" (Damasio 61).

23. Zuckow-Goldring and Arbib studied the case of an infant who has seen an orange peeled many times and wishes to perform the same action. However, "she needs her mother's help to learn the sequence of grasps and directed actions entailed in orange peeling" in order to begin practicing the activity herself (2188). Assisted embodied experimentation is key to the learning of this skill—force, direction, maneuvering hand, orange, and (possibly also) peeler cannot be gauged through observation alone.

24. In the summer of 1988 the playwright, director and cast of *Our Country's Good* went to see a performance of Howard Baker's *The Love of a Good Man* performed by prisoners serving life sentences. Wertenbaker describes this "unforgettable evening" as one which was "pivotal for the acting and writing of *Our Country's Good*: it confirmed all our feelings about the power and value of theatre." Some months later, Wertenbaker was invited to see a production her play at Bludston. (Program for the production at The Young Vic Theatre, October 22, 1998, directed by Max Stafford-Clark, prefaced by the playwright. There are no page numbers for the exchange of letters discussed below).

25. Preface to the play, June 1991, rpt. Methuen student edition 1995.

26. Walker does not refer to *Our Country's Good* but discusses Megan Terry's 1966 play *Viet Rock*, in which actors slip between portraying both Americans and Vietnamese in the same scene.

27. Once again, this is Wertenbaker's invention. In the novel Ralph is allowed all the actors he needs. Moreover, Arscott is not the one to escape but rather Caesar, who has no part in the play.

28. As mentioned above, the audiences of the original 1988 London production coincided with a revival of *The Recruiting Officer*. Audiences inspired by Wertenbaker to see Farquhar were invited to do so the very next evening. Moreover, because the same actors acted in both plays, further extending the playful doubling of roles discussed above, one could almost imagine that the latter production was indeed the convict-play left out of *Our Country's Good*. A *further* doubling occurred on the occasion of the company traveling with the play to Australia. While the British actors were double-billing *Our Country's Good* and *The Recruiting Officer* in Sydney, half a mile from the original penal colony, The Melbourne Theatre Company were doing the same in Melborne (Carlson 279).

29. The novel, on the contrary, recognizes that despite the success of the play, the subsequent lives of the vast majority of its participants were tragic. However, those who served out their sentence and made a new life in Australia usually prospered and the historical Sideway really did open a playhouse. Others, like Dabby, managed to escape but did not survive the voyage back. Ralph, having been sent by the military to other postings, was fatally wounded and died on the same day as his son at St. Nicole Mole. Although the harsh realities of eighteenth-century life do not allow the convicts to benefit from all they have learned to the extent the readers/audience might wish, they nevertheless stand before us as a mark of the tremendous capacity of the soul for rejuvenation and the possibilities opened up by engaged empathy.

30. The historical Captain Tench actually describes Thomas Barret, executed for theft while his accomplices were mercifully pardoned, as "an old and desperate offender, who died with that hardy spirit, which too often is found in the worst and most abandoned class of men" (Tench 74/44).

31. The manuscript (1789) claims on the title page to be "compiled from authentic papers," which there is no reason to doubt, and features drawings, maps and letters from a number of officers, but is highly unlikely to have been written by Phillip, particularly as it is written in the third person and praises him so copiously, a measure of immodesty that does not seem to fit descriptions of Phillip's character. James J. Auchmuty, the editor of the printed version of *The Voyage* (Sydney: Angus and Robertson, 1970) writes, "it is extremely doubtful if Phillip knew in advance that his reports from the new colony were to be the basis of a commercial publication" (ix). The name of the editor is unknown but the book is commissioned and compiled by John Stockwell of Piccadilly publishers eager to satisfy public demand for exciting tales of adventures overseas mixing actual discoveries and news with macabre tales and miraculous events. He describes Phillip as "one of the greatest British sea Captains...firm and courageous, lonely yet sympathetic, he laid the foundations of a British dominion in the Southern Seas whose development still continues..." (xiii), but no accounts suggest that he was an outstanding social reformer.

32. In his *An account of the English colony in New South Wales* (1789), the historical Captain Collins describes at length the kind of assistance provided to a convict who had completed his sentence and wished to become a settler. His training as a farmer and his desire to work the land were met with the allotment of two acres on which a hut was built for him. Not only was Phillip interested in rewarding his industrious and honest habits, "holding out encouragement to such dispositions" but, in addition, the governor "was desirous of trying, by his means, in what time an industrious active man, with certain assistance, would

be enabled to support himself in this country as a settler" (Collins 75). The free settler is therefore furnished with "tools and implements of husbandry," grain, stock and other help. This indicates a policy of helping those who help themselves and of perceiving the convicts—once freed—as full citizens of the new colony.

33. Amidst the causes of mortality in the colony, writes Tench, "excessive toil and a scarcity of food are not to be numbered, as the reader will easily conceive, when informed, that they have the same allowance of provisions as every officer and soldier in the garrison; and are indulged by being exempted from labor every Saturday afternoon and Sunday. On the latter of these days they are expected to attend divine service..." (Tench 136/72).

34. Locke declares that "God gave the world to men in common" (1689: v.34: 114)—and so each man should have his fair share. His definition of property begins with one's own body: "every man has a property in his own person: this nobody has any right to but himself" (1689: V. 27: 111) and extends to further property, whether inherited or earned through labor. This is also new to the convicts.

35. Of course, as Richard Ashcraft points out, Locke was writing this with the hope that readers would recognize Charles II and later James II as tyrants, justifying resistance, even rebellion (Ashcraft 1994: 234).

36. The play also discusses a third kind of contract—the contract of love between Mary and Ralph.

37. This is related to, but distinct from, Locke's notion of the "public will" expressed in the laws of the nation and to which the ruler is bound (1689: xiii.151: 167). Rousseau's theories have since been criticized for their potentially dangerous justification of the enforcement of conformity: "whoever refuses to obey the general will shall be compelled to do so by the whole body. This means nothing else than he will be forced to be free"...(177). This danger is explored in the novel but not in the play.

38. In the First Treatise, Locke refers to a "Compact" between individuals (I.iv.43: 188).

39. By using the term "sovereign" to denote the power of the collective, Rousseau transfers power from the prince to the people. He also annihilates the logic of civil defiance because civic duty and personal interest become indistinguishable. Indeed the date of the convict productions is, as noted above, 1789, the year of The French Revolution. An element of irony may have been attached to the historic viceroy's putting on a play in the King's honor at a location so remote from the King that he may never learn of the gesture, at the same time as the monarchy in France was deposed, but as the king's birthday was on June 4th, and as there had been no supply ship for months before that date so that the colony was in danger of starvation (*Country* 17), it is unlikely the governor had received news of the revolution.

40. Unlike Hobbes' ruler, who assumes absolute power, Locke claimed that the people have a right to resist their ruler if he is tyrannical. Tyranny is defined thus: "when the governor, however entitled, makes not the law, but his will, the rule; and his commands and actions are not directed to the preservation of the properties of his people, but the satisfaction of his own ambition, revenge, covetousness, or any other irregular passion," that is "his own private, separate advantage" (1689: xviii.199: 188). In other words, the ruler develops "an interest distinct from that of the public" (1689: xiv.164 : 173). Ironically, though Ross expects cooperative government to encourage mutiny, this is precisely what Locke would expect to prevent mutiny—an indeed it did.

41. This claim of course resonates powerfully with Cavell and Spolsky's conception of "good enough", detailed in Chapter 1.

42. It cannot be denied that the colony assumes power over the local Aboriginal population and that the expansionist plans of the British Empire later have devastating effects upon the Aboriginal people. However, the fact that the Aborigine is only present as distant on-looker in the play, though by the end he has caught small pox—a hint at the destructive effect colonialization will have upon his people and their culture—does not mean he has been marginalized. In fact, by casting the aboriginal, didgeridoo-playing Tom E. Lewis for this part in the Melbourne (1989) production of the play, the character of the native was perceived by Australian reviewers as "the absolute through line" of the play, "unavoidably about the power impositions of coloni-zation" (O'Donnell, MTC Program cited in Carlson). As well as tak-ing into account the necessary brevity required by the genre of drama, one must credit Wertenbaker with trying to re-introduce the element of race into her play by having the black, pagan Caesar take part in the convict-production, which he does not in the novel. She also leaves out his ignominious conduct in the novel—incontrollable appetites, theft, and women battery—making him a far more sympathetic char-acter. Moreover, because of her own multicultural and multi-lingual background—born in Canada (1951), educated in France and Greece, long-term resident of the UK—it would be simply ignorant to sug-gest Wertenbaker wishes to enforce homogeneity. As for Wilson's cen-tral complaint about Wertenbaker erasing the irony attached to the Governor's speech regarding theatre being "an expression of civiliza-tion" (*Country* 9) it is quite clearly mistaken in my view. Wilson ignores the fact that Phillip and H. E. have many discrepancies. The theatre-advocate who makes this speech in the play does not have a pet-native, while H. E., the viceroy in the novel, does not make speeches about the redemptive power of drama.Finally, I must also take issue with Wilson's complaint that the Governor in Wertenbaker's play is stripped of the homoerotic relationship with the captive aboriginal Arabanoo so that we are denied the psychological and political implications of the

captive loving his captor and the native dressing in colonial clothes. In *The Playmaker*, H. E.'s plan to capture a native, "quickly turning him into a gentlemen ambassador back to his own people" (Keneally 28) is considered a "strange enthusiasm" and his over-zealous attachment to the native Arabanoo progressively becomes the source of ridicule as well as malicious rumours. But H. E. is presented as a man of contrasts. He is by nature a recluse, a quiet, contemplative, unimposing man and yet both a brave soldier and a capable leader. His comprehension of the brutality of this capture may be incomplete, but those who know him, like Davy and Harry, are certain he has only fatherly affections towards the native and seeks no personal satisfaction or gains (160). Ralph too is convinced that H. E. would never consider abusing Arabanoo, even if he were homosexual, which is thoroughly questionable. In conclusion, most readers of *The Playmaker* likely sympathize with Ralph's discomfort, agreeing that abusing the *ab origines'* trust and capturing one of them, as well as enforced enculturation, is "a violation" (170), but this is not of a sexual nature.

43. In performance, the audience is also "recruited" to this point of view by the staging of this scene. In both Royal Court productions, this scene was enacted with the actors' backs presented to the audience so that the audience joined them in their backstage excitement and anticipation. Apparently the Melbourne production chose to have the actors face the audience, perhaps implicating them in potential colonization (see also Carlson 285).

44. Captain Tench mentions this prologue in his journal but makes no suggestion of subversion: "Some of the actors acquitted themselves with great spirit, and received the praises of the audience: a prologue and an epilogue, written by one of the performers, were also spoken on the occasion; which although not worth inserting here, contained some tolerable allusions to the situation of the parties, and the novelty of the stage-representation in New South Wales" (26/152).

45. In the novel, as I have mentioned, the play is performed before a mass gathering of the entire colony—convicts and officers. This did not happen in reality. Convicts were not invited to the historical performance.

46. It is encouraging to note that the historical Sideway indeed founded his own theatre when he was emancipated (Keneally 360).

47. see especially *TMS* Part VI section III—of Self-Command.

48. Smith's economic theory states that "commerce and manufactures," that is, the rise of influence and prosperity of the industrial towns of Europe and the subsequent trade with the countryside, is responsible for having "introduced order and good government, and with them, the liberty and security of individuals, among the inhabitants of the country", thereby freeing them from "servile dependency upon their superiors" (1776: III.iv 508). Opulence, as he calls it, has led to a just

system of naturally self-regulated give-and-take bartering, "nobody"— no one body or body of people—having "sufficient power to disturb" the operations of government " (1776: III.iv 514). "A revolution of the greatest importance to the public happiness was in this manner brought about by two different orders of people who had not the least intention of serving the public," bringing about, by default of the pursuit of self-interest directed by market forces, "the cause and occasion of the improvement and cultivation of the country" (515).

49. He also notes that the concept of individual liberty may be traced back to Luther's Reformation, and yet most of the revolutions that took place from that time on aimed to attain civic, rather than personal, liberty.

50. Reddy argues that, after 1794, a collective cover-up ensued, by which the role of emotions in past decades was also denied, as part of the need to re-evaluate the very basis of moral and political theory (Reddy 2000: 110). It is certainly the case that, as the nineteenth century unfolded, the trend was towards ever greater control, containment and curtailment of emotions and impulses, a preference for culture over any notion of natural instinctual responses, and a strict (Evangelical) moral code that stifled natural feelings—generating a range of pathologies born of repression.

51. In the transcript of the famous August 4th National Assembly, at which the French formulated the initial draft of the *Rights of Man*, expressions such as "humanitarian" considerations, "patriotic sacrifices," and "selfless" benevolent motives are rife (Reddy 134). Delegates voted against privileges which they themselves enjoyed, in good faith that this was advantageous to the collective, and the atmosphere of increasing (hour by hour) "spontaneous acts of generosity" spurred voters to set aside calculating the details of legislative reform and allow themselves to be swept up by a tide of fraternal sentiments (Reddy 135).This indicates the extent to which the delegates were motivated by (group-generated) emotional overflow and the approbation of such overflow. By 1802, Wordsworth, celebrating emotional overflow, would restrict its expression to the production of poetry, but in pre-revolution France it seems to have been prominent.

4   "A Spiritual Dance:" Moisés Kaufman's *33 Variations*

1. *33 Variations* has not, to date, been published. I am not certain of the reasons for this delay as I saw it at the Eugene O'Neill Theatre in New York in February 2008, with Jane Fonda in the lead as Katherine Brandt, Samantha Mathis as Clara, Colin Hanks as Mike, Susan Kellermann as Gertie, and Zach Grenier as Beethoven. The citations in this chapter, therefore, are from the script manuscript

entitled "Draft 03-03-2009", kindly provided by Dramatists Play Services, Inc. A "spiritual dance" is Katherine's phrase, 33V: 124.

2. Naturally, this connects to the discussion of art as a conduit to immortality in Chapter 2 of this book.

3. In 1797, while living in Alfoxden, a neighbour of Coleridge's by the name of John Cruikshank related a strange dream he had had about "a skeleton ship." This was only the initial impetus of course, but it did inspire the epic ballad (see Gardner 1965: 18–19).

4. As the pre-Socratic philosopher Heraclitus famously said: "You cannot step twice into the same river."

5. For an introduction to Language of the Birds and other occult and mystic teachings, see Walker 1995.

6. As the extensive discussion of basic and moral emotions in Chapter 3 already explained, basic emotions include: fear, happiness, surprise, sadness, anger and disgust.

7. In *Aspects of the Novel* (1927) E. M. Forster wrote that "In daily life we never understand each other, neither complete clairvoyance nor complete confessional exists. We know each other approximately, by external signs, and these serve well enough as a basis for society And even for intimacy. But people in a novel can be understood completely by the reader, if the novelist wishes; their inner as well as their outer life can be exposed. And this is why they often seem more definite than characters in history, or even our own friends; we have been told all about them that can be told" (1927: 54–55).

8. In Sartre's famous discussion in *Being and Nothingness* of the *look* or *gaze,* he describes a hypothetical situation in which he (or any man) is peeping at someone through a keyhole. At first, he is caught up in the situation; he is in a pre-reflexive state in which his entire consciousness is directed at the action taking place in the room into which he is peeping. But, suddenly, he hears a floorboard creak behind him, and he becomes immediately ashamed of his transgressive behaviour: "I shudder as a wave of shame sweepes over me. Somebody has seen me" (Sartre 1943: 339). At this moment, he automatically sees himself through the eyes of the Other observing him. The impression of being observed (and, thus, objectified) can be either real or imagined. As Freud argued with regard to the superego, it requires no "real" external correlative. Our experience of the *look* is subjective— it constitutes our idea of, and response to, how we imagine the Other perceives us. Once the notion of "being-as-object" is planted in one's consciousness, one cannot return to a pre-reflexive state; whether or not one is being observed, one is "already in the state of being-looked-at" (1943: 340).

9. Recent cognitive neuroscience research, as detailed in Gallace and Spence's review of the current status of findings, holds that the brain differentiates between the more affective aspects of touch and

affectively-neutral tactile sensations (someone stroking one's check with affection, vs. brushing against a doorframe by mistake). The neural correlates of the more affective aspects of tactile processing have also suggested that the insular cortex might be an important component of a system responsible for our emotional, hormonal, and affiliative responses to tactile contact between individuals engaged in behaviors such as social grooming and nurturing. The insular cortex is now thought to contribute to the processing of convergent signals arising from different sensory channels, to produce an emotionally relevant response to a given sensory experience. Thus, hypothesize Gallace and Spence, one might reasonably argue that "the neural network responsible for the processing of certain emotional aspects of tactile experiences is actually shared with the network responsible for processing information from other sensory modalities" and that "the more emotional aspects of tactile sensations may be also related to the functioning of the neural systems responsible for our memory of tactile sensations (2010: 252).

10. As discussed at length in the introduction to this book, empathy is, first and foremost, an involuntary physical response and should not be confused with sympathy. Indeed, Singer and colleagues' research into pain-related responses demonstrate that empathic experience "does not involve activation of an entire pain matrix, but only of that component associated with the affective dimension of pain experience." Moreover, in contrast to accounts of emotional contagion, they suggest that empathic responses can be "elicited automatically in the absence of an emotional cue (such as facial emotional expressions) through mere presentation of an arbitrary cue that signals the feeling state of another person" (1158). This becomes all the more pronounced when the family love-ties between pain-experiencer and observer are strong. However, it must be emphasized again that empathetic responses to pain need not result in automatic sympathy.

11. Henricson et al. recount studies that showed women with diabetes experienced blood glucose decreases after tactile touch, studies that showed women during the latent phase of labor could relax and recover their strength after tactile massage and studies that showed patients with anorexia nervosa felt a sense of relaxation and relief after tactile treatment. Furthermore, women with breast cancer experienced reduced nausea after the treatment and patients with a stroke made clear progress in terms of reduced incontinence, improved mobility and hygiene when they received tactile massage. None of the studies reported any negative effects of the treatment (Henricson et al. 2009: 324).

12. Initially, explain Henriscson et al., "the touch therapist prepares the room; lights are dimmed; soft relaxing music is played; curtains are drawn to provide privacy; towels are prepared in a heating cabinet

and staff are encouraged to keep the environment as quiet as possible. During tactile touch, the patient's body is wrapped in towels so they will not feel cold or be unnecessarily exposed. Only the part of the patient's body that is being touched is uncovered. To achieve positive effects, patients need repeated treatment for at least 30 minutes" (Henricson et al. 2009: 324).

13. Haidt claims that recent research "shows that there are some things worth striving for; there are external conditions of life that can make you lastingly happier. One of these conditions is relatedness—the bonds we form, and need to form, with others" (Haidt 2006: xii). Happiness requires a balance between inner and outer. Stoic asceticism may be a good defense mechanism against frustration and disappointment, but it also extinguishes the possibility of genuine happiness.

14. I discuss this theory at length in "Constructing Cognitive Scaffolding through Embodied Receptiveness: Toni Morrison's *The Bluest Eye*". *Style* 41.4 (2008): 385–408.

15. Naturally, severe burning would disallow any physical contact. But that is not to say that the injured individual no longer longs for that contact.

16. I refer the reader back to the discussion of mirror neurons and, in particular, Damasio's CDZs, in the introduction to this book.

17. Though Katherine's experiences in *33 Variations* can in no way be compared to the Nazi death camps, Consonni's ideas are pertinent here because of her attention to the ontological effects of continual and increasing pain and an existence hijacked by a steady movement towards, and anticipation of, death.

18. In *A Brief History of Time*, Stephen Hawking asserts that "We must accept that time is not completely separate from and independent of space, but is combined with it to form an object called space-time" (Hawking 1995: 24). He sees three time's arrows—the cosmological, the thermodynamic and the psychological; the third acting as a mediator between phenomenology and physics.

19. The term "multiverse" refers to the hypothetical set of multiple possible universes (including the historical universe we consistently experience) that together comprise everything that exists: space, time, matter, and energy, as well as the physical laws and constants that describe them. Philosopher and psychologist William James coined the term in 1895. The various universes within the multiverse are sometimes called parallel, alternative or quantum universes, and have been the object of studies and theories in cosmology, physics, astronomy, philosophy, psychology and fiction. Physics and cosmology professor Max Tegmark has provided a taxonomy of universes beyond the familiar observable universe. According to his calcification, the multiverse is divided into levels; each subsequent level encompasses

and expands the previous levels. Tegmark argues that, implausible as this may first seem, the existence of parallel universes, and also identical other selves in those universes, is highly likely, since "the simplest and most popular cosmological model today predicts that this [parallel] person actually exists in a Galaxy about $10^{10^{29}}$ meters from here. This does not even assume speculative modern physics, merely that space is infinite and rather uniformly filled with matter as indicated by recent astronomical observations. Your *alter ego* is simply a prediction of the so-called concordance model of cosmology, which agrees with all current observational evidence and is used as the basis for most calculations and simulations presented at cosmology conferences. In contrast, alternatives such as a fractal universe, a closed universe and a multiply connected universe have been seriously challenged by observations" (2003: 1). Tegmark asserts further that "it is becoming increasingly clear that multiverse models grounded in modern physics can in fact be empirically testable, predictive and falsifiable. [...] the key question is not whether there is a multiverse [...] but rather how many levels it has" (2003: 1). More recently, Robles-Perez and colleagues have suggest "a third-quantization" procedure that may effectively represent "a manyuniverse system" quantum mechanically. Such a manyuniverse system, they explain, can describe "either a multiverse made up of parent universes or a spacetime foam formed by popping baby Universes" (2010: 3).

20. Materialism does not entail determinism. The notion that individual humans and the world at large are made of the same atoms does not collapse the distinction between the external world and ourselves. If there is, and I agree with Clark that there is indeed a continual symbiotic relationship between brain-in-body and world, that still does not entail total merger. There must be a distinction between the two in order for agency to exist.

21. In contrast to Leontes, Katherine, like Paulina, acknowledges that close knowledge of a person's character is usually a valid consideration in the interpretation of their potential motivations. Indeed, Bonn in no way resembles Shakespeare's coast of Bohemia, yet when Katherine arrives there, her first email to Clara states: "Here I don't feel sick at all. The city exudes music" (33V: "BONN": 27). Beethoven's precious notebooks are kept underground, in a vast, windowless dungeon, guarded as fiercely as a high-security prison (presumably also symbolising Katherine's subconscious fears and desires); yet the notebooks are made of honey, and their chief warden swiftly transforms from prison-guard to guardian-angel. The hospital's examination room is in every way antithetical to the pastoral "green-world," yet in it Katherine hallucinate Beethoven, who provides her with comfort, both by validating her academic theories and

by supporting her body with his. Finally, physical therapy induces profound emotional and spiritual change, correcting Katherine's imbalance; teaching her the values traditionally associated with the pastoral genre, and enabling her to connect with her daughter, as Leontes connects with his at the end of *The Winter's Tale*. I am not suggesting that Kaufman intended these parallels so much as indicating that, in addition to sharing a disregard for strictly realistic plot devices, the plays share many themes, chief among them faith in embodied methods of communication.

22. Katherine does not suggest this but, perhaps, for Beethoven, there may have been a connection to the fact that Jesus died at 33?
23. This movement has become the official anthem of the European Union. Before that, it was famously incorporated into the plot of Stanley Kubrick's 1971 movie "A Clockwork Orange."
24. Dating as far back as 1809, we find notes of musical ideas which will be later used for this symphony. The material he gathered was ultimately used between 1822–1824 when the great symphony was elaborated" http://www.all-about-beethoven.com/symphony9.html
25. For instance, Clara complains to Mike that "there are no medicines, no treatment, no nothing" to help her mother. "Am I missing something?" (33V: "THE SKETCHES – PART 1" p.32). Mike describes Katherine's ailment as "an orphan disease": it is too rare to interest the pharmaceutical companies. Katherine does not expect Clara to mother her orphan, indeed she tries to evade Clara, but Clara assumes the role of caretaker. This is already something. When Katherine, after being hospitalized following a fall says "Nothing to worry about," (33V: "DANCING" p.52) she means yes, I am slowly decaying; there is no point in worrying about the inevitable. This does not make it nothing—it makes it a void which can be filled with whichever meaning is inserted into the term—this is where Katherine insists on taking control of the interpretation and significance of her decay.
26. Fonda's voice in the Broadway production of this scene has been described as "heartbreaking in its reedy frailness" (Brantley 2009).
27. She tells Nelly of a dream she had in which she had gone to heaven, but "heaven did not seem to be my home; and I broke my heart with weeping to come back to earth; and the angels were so angry they flung me out into the middle of the heath on the top of Wuthering Heights, where I woke sobbing for joy" (Brontë 1847: 80).
28. This does not apply to many melodramas and farces.
29. Kaufman is of Jewish descent. Throughout Kufman's manuscript, God is spelt G_d, suggesting that he is, to some extent at least, a believer. However, I do not know the extent to which he is observant and I do not believe it to be relevant here.

30. Indeed, Coleridge's "conversation poems" are all pertinent here because of their connection to the theme of variations, through close modelling upon Hartley's "Doctrine of Vibrations" and "Doctrine of Associations" by which he hypothesized how complex constellations of associative thought are produced—just like a series of variations on a theme. Moreover, Coleridge's poems connect also to the theme of a commoners' waltz: Blank verse is distinguished by having a regular meter but no rhyme. In English, blank verse is also the meter that most closely resembles common speech patterns. Thus, it is not attempting to be elevated above but, rather, grounded in, everyday interaction. Conversational lyrics by "a man speaking to men." Further yet, Beethoven produced a series of "conversation notebooks." At first, when Beethoven finally lost his hearing, his interlocutors would write down their remarks and he would speak his reply. Thus, the notebooks that survive, record only half of the conversation: what others said, but not his response, just like Coleridge's poems. After that, as discussed below, Beethoven learned to lipread.

31. "Freude trinken alle Wesen / An den Bresten der Natur"

32. The Aeolian harp is an instrument constructed of strings stretched across an oblong box with a central sound cavity. Each string, although the same length, is of different thickness, and all are tuned to a single tone. The instrument is then placed in a breezy location, such as an open window, and is played upon by the wind—or Aeolis, God of the wind—causing a harmonic vibration, the pitch and intensity of which varies with wind speed.

33. Hartley's "Doctrine of Vibrations" describes the intimate connection of physiological and psychical facts, believing that sensation is the result of a vibration of the minute particles of the medullary substance of the nerves. His "Doctrine of Associations" hypothesizes that the course of reminiscence and of the thoughts generally, is accounted for by the existence of vibrations in the brain. The nature of these vibrations is determined both by each man's past experience and by the circumstances of the moment, which causes one or another tendency to prevail over the rest. Sensations are often grouped together, becoming associated with the ideas corresponding to other associative matrices, and the ideas corresponding to these associated sensations are further connected to one another in extending patterns. Though his theory was not accurate in terms of current neurobilogical findings, it does correspond in many ways to the understanding of neural clusters and interconnected networks described in the introduction to this book.

34. "den grossen Ring"

35. Audiences, sitting in their seats, are necessarily removed frown the stage action, observing it from a distance. And yet, as argued

throughout this book, the multifaceted power of drama to engage the spectator on every level of Being, renders the experience one of dynamic participation. In this participation inhere both conscious, involved alertness and involuntary physical simulation.

36. For centuries, philosophers have grappled with the problem of consciousness, what it may be, how it arises, whether or not it is produced by material elements, such as brain cells, and how it contributes to the production of thoughts and feelings. Interesting as this question is, it is not the focus of the present study. However, it is useful to note that the vast majority of both cognitive scientists and philosophers today are convinced that consciousness arises from brain functions: "the present task in the neurobiology of consciousness is to explain exactly how brain processes create consciousness" (Searle 2011: 52). As John Searle explains: "to be fully conscious you have to have three features: (1) to be awake, (2) to have an operational mind, and (3) to have the sense of self as a protagonist of the experience" (2011: 51). According to Jonathan Kramnick, the notion that consciousness is tethered to the material of the brain goes back at least as far as Lucretius. He already supposed that not only physical but mental phenomena may be predicted by the laws of atomic motion. Kramnick's analysis is pertinent to this study because he claims that "Every mental event that is causally tied to a physical event is in virtue of this connection a physical event. [...] Thinking is itself a kind of action and action a kind of thought, each the echo of the other in a world made only of atoms" (Kramnick 2011: 17).

Conclusion

1. Gordon makes a clear distinction between "total projection," which is simple, situational and immediate, (for instance, when our fellow hiker turns pale and shouts "run away!") and "partial projection," which is more personal and may involve adjustments to our worldview or a reconsideration of our perspective, even consideration of deviant (to our mind) behavior (Gordon 1995: 103).

2. Rokotnitz, Naomi. "Too far gone in disgust": Mirror Neurons and the Manipulation of Embodied Responses in *The Libertine*." *Configurations* 16:3 (2010) 400–426.

Works Cited

Agnew, Zaharina K., Kishore K. Bhakoo, Basant K. Puri. "The Human Mirror System: A Motor Resonance Theory of Mind-Reading." *Brain Research Review* 54 (2007): 286–293.

Arbib, Michael A. "From monkey-like action recognition to human language: an evolutionary framework for neuroliguistics." *Behavioural Brain Sciences* 28 (2005): 105–124.

Arbib Michael A. and Mary B. Hesse. *The Construction of Reality.* Cambridge: Cambridge UP, 1986.

Ashcraft, Richard. "Locke's Political Philosophy." *The Cambridge Companion to Locke.* ed. Vere Chappell. Cambridge: Cambridge UP, 1994.

Auvray, Malika., Alberto Gallace, Hong Z. Tan and Charles Spence. "Crossmodal Change Blindness Between Vision and Touch." *Acta Psychologica* 126 (2007): 79–97.

Avrahami, Einat. *The Invading Body: Reading Illness Autobiographies.* Charlottesville and London: U of Virginia P, 2007.

Badiou, Alain and Nina Power. "Existence and Death." *Discourse* 24.1 (2002): 63–73.

Barroll, J. Leeds. *Artificial Persons: The Formation of Character in the Tragedies of Shakespeare.* Columbia UP, 1974.

Berlin, Isaiah. *Two Concepts of Liberty.* Oxford: Oxford UP, 1958.

Bloom, Harold. *The Anxiety of Influence: A Theory of Poetry.* 2nd ed. New York: Oxford UP, 1997.

Bloom, Paul. *Descartes' Baby.* (First published 2004 by William Heinemann). London: Arrow Books, 2005.

Borenstein, Elhanan and Eytan Ruppina. "The Evolution of Imitation and Mirror Neurons in Adaptive Agents." *Cognitive Systems Research* 6.3 (2005): 229–242.

Bradshaw, Jon. "Tom Stoppard, Nonstop" (1977). *Tom Stoppard In Conversation.* ed. Paul Delaney. Ann Arbor: U of Michigan P, 1994. 89–99.

Brantley, Ben. "Beethoven and Fonda: Broadway Soul Mates." Theatre Review. *The NY Times.* March 10 2009. http://theater.nytimes.com /2009/03/10/theater/reviews/10thir.html

Brendel, Alfred. "Beethoven's Diabelli Variations." *Alfred Brendel On Music*. Chicago Review P, 2001. Cited http://en.wikipedia.org/wiki/Diabelli_Variations#cite_note-4

Brontë, Emily. *Wuthering Heights* (1847). London: Penguin, 1994.

Butler, Judith. *Gender Trouble: Feminism and the Subversion of Identity*. New York: Routledge, 1990.

Brook, Andrew and Robert J. Stainton. *Knowledge and Mind: A Philosophical Introduction*. Cambridge, MA: MIT Press, 2000.

Bynum, Caroline. "Why All the Fuss about the Body? A Medievalist's Perspective." *Critical Inquiry* 22 (1995): 1–33.

Carlson, Susan. "Issues of Identity, Nationality and Performance: the Reception of Two Plays by Timberlake Wertenbaker." *New Theatre Quarterly* 9.35 (1993): 267–289.

Carruthers, Peter, and Peter Smith, eds. *Theories of Theories of Mind*. Cambridge: Cambridge UP, 1996.

Carroll, Lewis. *Alice's Adventures in Wonderland, Through The Looking Glass, The Hunting of the Snark*. (Originally published in order: 1865, 1872, 1876). London: The Bodley Head, 1963.

Cavell, Stanley. *Must We Mean What We Say?* Cambridge: Cambridge UP, 1969.

———. *The Claim of Reason: Wittgenstein, Skepticism, Morality and Tragedy*. New York: Oxford UP, 1979.

———. *Disowning Knowledge In Six Plays of Shakespeare*. Cambridge: Cambridge UP, 1987.

Chaillet, Ned. "Wertenbaker Timberlake." *Contemporary Dramatics*. 4th ed. Ed. D. L. Kirkpatrick. London: St. James P, 1988. 554.

Check Hayden, Erika. "Life is Complicated." *Nature* 46.4 (2010): 664–667.

Clark, Andy. "Where Brain, Body and Mind Collide." *Daedalus* 127.2 (1998): 247–280.

———. *Natural-Born Cyborgs: Minds, Technologies and the Future of Human Intelligence*. New York: Oxford UP, 2003.

———. "Language, Embodiment, and the Cognitive Niche." *Trends in Cognitive Sciences* 10.8 (2006): 370–374.

Clark, Ralph. *The Journal and Letters of Lt. Ralph Clark 1787–1792*. eds. Paul G. Fidlon and R. J. Ryan. Australian Documents Library, Netley.

Colebrook, Clare. "Questioning Representation." *SubStance* 29.2 (2000): 47–67.

Coleridge, Samuel Taylor. *Biographia Literaria: Or Biographical Sketches of My Literary Life and Opinions* (1817). *The Collected Works of Samuel Taylor Coleridge*. Eds. James Engell and W. Jackson Bate. Princeton UP, 1983.

Collins, David. *An Account of the English Colony in New South Wales*. Ed. Brian H. Fletcher. Sydney: A. H. & A. W. Reed, 1975.

Connerton, Paul. *How Societies Remember*. Cambridge: Cambridge UP, 1989.

Consonni, Manuella. "Primo Levi, Robert Antelme, and the Body of the Muselmann." *Partial Answers* 7.2 (2009): 423–259.

———. "Semantic Shift and the Experience of Pain." *Presentation at Scholion: Knowledge and Pain Conference.* Hebrew University of Jerusalem, May 2010.

Cooke, John William. "The Optical Allusion: Perception and Form in Stoppard's *Travesties.*" *Modern Drama* 24 (1981): 525–539.

Corrigen, Robert W., ed. *Tragedy: Vision and Form.* San Francisco: Chandler, 1965.

———. "Tragicomedy." *The World of The Theatre.* Glenview: Scott, Foresman. (1979). Rpt. in *Comedy Meaning and Form,* 2nd ed. Ed. Robert W. Corrigen. New York: Harper & Row, 1981. 222–228.

Cromwell, Howard Casey and Jaak Panksepp. "Rethinking the Cognitive Revolution from a Neural Perspective: How overuse/misuse of the term 'cognition' and the neglect of affective controls in behavioral neuroscience could be delaying progress in understanding the BrainMind." In press for *Neuroscience and Biobehavioral Reviews* (2011).

Damasio, Antonio. *The Feeling of What Happens: Body and Emotion in the Making of Consciousness.* New York and London: Harcourt, 1999.

Damasio, Antonio and Kasper Meyer. "Behind the Looking-Glass". *Nature* 454 (2008): 167–168.

Davey, Graham C. L., Steve Bickerstaffe, and B. A. MacDonald. "Experienced Disgust Causes a Negative Interpretation Bias: a Causal Role for Disgust in Anxious Psychopathology." *Behaviour Research and Therapy* 44 (2006): 1375–1384.

Decety, Jean. "To What Extent Is the Experience of Empathy Mediated by Shared Neural Circuits?" *Emotion Review* (2010): 1–4.

Decety Jean, Julie Grezes, N. Costes, Daniela Perani, Marc Jeannerod, Emanuel Procyk, Fondazione Paolo Grassi, and Ferrucio Fazio. "Brain Activity During Observation of Actions: Influence of Action Content and Subject's Strategy." *Brain* 120 (1997): 1763–1777.

Delaney, Paul, ed. *Tom Stoppard in Conversation.* Ann Arbor: U of Michigan P, 1994. 103-106.

Derrida, Jacques. "Structure, Sign, and Play in the Discourse of the Human Sciences." *The Structuralist Controversy.* eds. Richard Macksey and Eugenio Donato. Baltimore: Johns Hopkins UP, 1970.

———. "Signature Event Context." *Glyph* 1 (1977): 172–179.

Dolan, Frances E. *Dangerous Familiars: Representations of Domestic Crime in England 1550–1700.* Ithaca: Cornell UP, 1994.

Duffy, Edward. "Stanley Cavell's Redemptive Reading: A Philosophical Labor in Progress." *Ordinary Language Criticism: Literary Thinking after Cavell after Wittgenstein.* Eds. Kenneth Dauber and Walter Jost. Evanston: Northwestern UP, 2003. 31–53.

Eagleman, David M. "Visual Illusions and Neurobiology." *Nature Reviews Neuroscience* 2 (2001): 920–926.

Eakin, Emily. "I Feel, Therefore I Am." *NY Times* April 19, 2003. http://www.nytimes.com/2003/04/19/books/i-feel-therefore-i-am.html? src=pm

Ekman, Paul. "Facial Expression of Emotion." *American Psychologist* 48 (1983): 384–392.

———. "An Argument for Basic Emotions." *Cognition and Emotion* 6 (1992): 169–200.

Eichelbaum, Stanley. "So Often Produced He Ranks with Shaw." *San Francisco Examiner* 28.3 (1977). Rpt. In full in *Tom Stoppard In Conversation*. ed. Paul Delaney. Ann Arbor: U of Michigan P, 1994. 103–106.

Fadiga, Luciano, Leonardo Fogassi, G. Pavesi, and Giacomo Rizolatti. "Motor Facilitation During Action Observation: a Magnetic Stimulation Study." *Journal of Neurophysiology* 73 (1995): 2608–2611.

Fadiga, Luciano and Vittorio Gallese. "Action Representation and Language in the Brain." *Theoretical Linguistics* 23 (1997): 267–280.

Field, Tiffany Martini. *Touch*. Cambridge, MA: MIT Press, 2001.

Fish, Stanley E. *Is There A Text in This Class? The Authority of Interpretive Communities*. Cambridge: Harvard UP, 1980.

Fogassi, Leonardo., Ferrari Francesco Pier, Benno Gesierich, Stefano Rozzi, Fabian Chersi, and Giacommo Rizzolatti. "Parietal Lobe: From Action Organization to Intention Understanding." *Science* 308 (2005): 662–667.

Forster, E.M. *Aspects of the Novel* (1927). NY: Harcourt, 1954.

Gadamar, Hans-Georg. "Goethe and Philosophy." *Humboldt Bucherei 3*. Leipzig: Volk und Buch Verlag, 1947. Rpt. in full Paslick, Robert H. Trans. and Int. *Literature And Philosophy in Dialogue: Essays in German Literary Theory by Hans-Georg Gadamar*. Albany: State U of New York P, 1994.

Gardener, Martin. Int. and notes. *The Annotated Ancient Mariner*. NY: Meridian Books, 1965.

Gallace, Alberto and Charles Spence. "The Science of Interpersonal Touch: An Overview." *Neuroscience and Biobehavioral Reviews* 34 (2010): 246–259.

Gallagher, Shaun. *How the Body Shapes the Mind*. Oxford UP, 2005.

Gallagher, Shaun and Dan Zahavi. *The Phenomenological Mind: An Introduction to Philosophy of Mind and Cognitive Science*. Abingdon and NY: Routledge, 2008.

Gallese Vittorio. "The 'Shared Manifold' Hypothesis: From Mirror Neurons to Empathy." *Journal of Consciousness Studies* 8 5–7 (2001): 33–50.

Gallese, Vittorio and Alvin Goldman. "Mirror Neurons and the Simulation Theory of Mind-Reading." *Trends in Cognitive Sciences* 2.12 (December 1998): 493–502.

Gallese, Vittorio, Christian Keysers, and Giacomo Rizzolatti. "A Unifying View of the Basis of Social Cognition." *Trends in Cognitive Science* 8.9 (2004): 396–403.

Gazzola, Valeria, Lisa Aziz-Zadeh, and Christian Keysers. "Empathy and the Somatotopic Auditory Mirror System in Humans." *Current Biology* 16 (2006): 1824–1829.

Gold, Margaret. "Who are the Dadas of *Travesties?*" *Modern Drama* 21 (1978): 59–66.

Gomel, Elana. *Postmodern Science Fiction and Temporal Imagination.* New York and London: Continuum International Publishing Group, 2010.

Gordon, Robert. "The Simulation Theory: Objections and Misconceptions." *Folk Psychology.* Eds. Martin Davies and Tony Stone. Oxford: Blackwell, 1995. 100–122.

———. "'Radical' Simulationism." *Theories of Theories of Mind.* Ed. Peter Caruthers and Peter Smith. Cambridge: Cambridge UP, 1996. 11–21.

Green, Robert. *Pandosto, or The Triumph of Time* (1588). Ed. Frank Kermode in Shakespeare, William. *The Winter's Tale* (1610–11). The Signet Classic Shakespeare. Gen. Ed. Sylvan Barnet, Harmondsworth: Penguin, 1963.

Greenblatt, Stephen J. "Sidney's Arcadia and the Mixed Mode." *Studies in Philosophy* 70.3 (1973): 269–78. Rpt. *Essential Articles for the Study of Sir Phillip Sidney.* Ed. Arthur F. Kinney. Hamden, Conn.: Archen Books, 1986.

———. "Invisible Bullets: Renaissance Authority and its Subversion." *Shakespearean Negotiations: The Circulation of Social Energy in Renaissance England.* Berkeley: U of California P, 1988.

Grèzes, Julie, Nicolas Costes, and Jean Decety. "Top-Down Effect of Strategy on the Perception of Human Biological Motion: a PET Investigation." *Cognitive Neuropsychology* 15: 6/7/8 (1998): 553–582.

Grice, H. Paul. "Logic and Conversation." *Syntax and Semantics. Vol III: Speech Acts.* Eds. Peter Cole and Jerry L. Morgan. New York: Academic P., 1975.

Grishakova, Marina. "Beyond the Frame: Cognitive Science, Common Sense and Fiction." *Narrative* 17.2 (May 2009): 162–187.

Haack, Susan. "Staying for an Answer: The Untidy Process of Groping for Truth." *TLS,* 9.7 July 9, 1999.

Habermas, Jürgen. "Modernity—an Incomplete Project." First published as "Modernity versus Post-modernity." *New German Critique* 22 (1981). Rpt. *Modernism/ Postmodernism.* Ed and int. Peter Brooker. London: Longman, 1992. 125–138.

Haidt, Jonathan. "The Moral Emotions." *Handbook of Affective Sciences.* Eds. R. J. Davidson, K. R. Scherer, HH Goldsmith. Oxford: Oxford UP, 2003. 862–870.

Haidt, Jonathan. *The Happiness Hypothesis.* London: Arrow Books, Random House, 2006.

Haidt, Jonathan, Clark MaCauley, and Paul Rozin. "Individual Differences in Sensitivity to Disgust: A Scale Sampling Seven Domains of Disgust Elicitors." *Personality and Individual Differences* 16 (1994): 701–713.

Hamann, Stephen. "Nosing In On The Emotional Brain." *Nature Neuroscience* 6.2 (2003): 106–108.

Hamilton, Donna B. "The Winter's Tale and the Language of Union, 1604–1611." *Shakespeare Studies* XXI (1993): 228–250.

Hart, F. Elizabeth. "Performance, Phenomenology, and the Cognitive Turn." *Performance and Cognition: Theatre Studies After the Cognitive Turn.* eds. F. E. Hart and B. McConachie. NY: Routledge, 2006.

Hatfield, Elaine, John T. Cacioppo, and Richard L. Rapson. "Emotional Contagion." *Studies in Emotion and Social Interaction.* Cambridge: Cambridge UP, 1994.

Hawkins, Harriet. *Likeness of Truth in Elizabethan and Restoration Comedy.* Oxford: Oxford UP, 1972.

Hawking, Stephen. *A Brief History Of Time: From Big Bang To Black Holes: From the Big Bang to Black Holes.* Bentam, 1995.

Hayles, Katherine N. *Chaos Bound: Orderly Disorder in Contemporary Literature and Science.* Ithaca: Cornell University Press, 1990.

———. ed., *Chaos and Order: Complex Dynamics in Literature and Science.* Chicago: U of Chicago P, 1991.

———. "The Materiality of Informatics." *Configurations* 1.1 (1993): 147–170.

Heidegger, Martin. *Being and Time* (1927). Trans. Joan Stambaugh. New York: NY State UP, 1996.

Henderson David and Terence Horgan. "Simulation and Epistemic Competence." In Hans Herbert Kögler and Karsten R. Steuber eds. and int. *Empathy and Agency.* Boulder: Westview, 2000. 119–141.

Henricson, Maria, Kerstin Segestena, Anna-Lena Berglund, and Sylivia Määttä. "Enjoying tactile touch and gaining hope when being cared for in intensive care—A phenomenological hermeneutical study." *Intensive and Critical Care Nursing* 25 (2009): 323–331.

Hickok, Gregory. "Eight Problems for the Mirror Neuron Theory of Action Understanding in Monkeys and Humans." *Journal of Cognitive Neuroscience* 21.7 (2009): 1229–1243.

Hobbes, Thomas. *Leviathan.* (1651). Oxford: Oxford UP (World's Classics), 1996.

Hosek, Jennifer Ruth and Walter J. Freeman. "Osmetic Ontogenesis, or Olfaction Becomes You: The Neurodynamic, Intentional Self and Its Affinities with the Foucaultian/Butlerian Subject." *Configurations* 9 (2001): 509–541.

Horace. *Ars Poetica.* Trans. E. H. Blakeney, in *Literary Criticism: Plato to Dryden.* Ed. Allen H. Gilbert. NY, 1940. 139.

Houghton, Walter E. "Character of the Age." In Richard A. Levine ed. *Backgrounds to Victorian Literature.* San Francisco: Chandler Publishing, 1967. 15–41.

Hudson, Roger, Cathrine Itzin, and Simon Trussler. "Abuses for the Audience: Towards a High Comedy of Ideas" (1974). Rpt. *Tom Stoppard In Conversation.* ed. Paul Delaney. Ann Arbor: U of Michigan P, 1994. 51–72.

Hunter, Robert Grams. *Shakespeare and The Comedy of Forgiveness.* New York: Columbia UP, 1965.

Hutcheon, Linda. *A Theory of Parody: The Teachings of Twentieth-Century Art Forms.* New York: Methuen, 1985.

Hytner, Nicholas. "Behold the Swelling Scene: The Theatrical Consequences of Shakespeare's Addiction to Truth." *TLS* 1.11 (2002): 22.

Iacoboni, Marco, Roger P. Woods, Marcel Brass, Harold Bekkering, John C. Maziotta, and Giacomo Rizzolatti. "Cortical Mechanisms of Human Imitation." *Science* 286 (1999): 2526–2528.

Inverso, Marybeth. "*Der Straf-block*: Performance and Execution in Barnes, Griffiths, and Wertenbaker." *Modern Drama* 36:3 (1993): 420–430.

Jackson, Tony E. "Literary Interpretation and Cognitive Literary Studies." *Poetics Today* 24.2 (2003): 191–205.

Johnson, Mark. *The Meaning of the Body: Aesthetics of Human Understanding.* Chicago: U of Chicago P, 2007.

Kagan, Jerome. "Unity of Knowledge: The Convergence of Natural and Human Science." *Annals of the New York Academy of Sciences* 935 (2001): 177–190.

Kaplan, Lindsay M. and Katherine Eggert, "Sexual Slander in *The Winter's Tale*." *Renaissance Drama* 25 (1994): 89–118.

Kaufman, Moisés. *33 Variations.* "Draft 03-03-2009." Dramatic Play Services Inc.

Keen, Suzanne. "A Theory of Empathy." *Narrative* 14.3 (2006): 207–236.

Kelly, Katherine E. "Tom Stoppard Journalist: Through the Stage Door." *Modern Drama* 33 (1990): 380–393.

Keneally, Thomas. *The Playmaker.* London: Hodder and Stoughton, 1987.

Keysers, Chrsitian, Bruno Wicker, Valeria Gazzola, Jean-Luc Anton, Leonardo Fugassi, and Vittorio Gallese. "A Touching Sight: SII/PV Activation During the Observation and Experience of Touch." *Neuron* 42 (2004): 335–346.

Keysers, Christian and Valeria Gazzola. "Integrating Simulation and Theory of Mind: From Self to social cognition." *Trends in Cognitive Science* 11.5 (2007): 194–196.

Kinderman, William. *Beethoven*, Oxford UP, 1995.

Kögler, Hans Herbert and Karsten R. Steuber. eds. and int. *Empathy and Agency.* Boulder: Westview, 2000.

Kohler, Evelyne, Christian Keyers, Maria Alessandra Umilta, Leonardo Fogassi, Vittorio Gallese, and Giacomo Rizolatti. "Hearing Sound, Understanding Actions: Action Representation in Mirror Neurons." *Science* 297.5582 (2002): 846–848.

Kramnick, Jonathan. "Against Literary Darwinism." *Critical Inquiry* 37 (2011): 315–347.

Kramnick, Jonathan. "Living with Lucretius." in Helen Deutsch and Mary Terrell, eds. *Vital Matters: Eighteenth-Century Views of Conception, Life, and Death.* Ann Arbor: U of Michigan P, 2011.

Krausz, Michael. Ed and int. *Relativism: Interpretation and Confrontation.* Notre Dame, Indiana: U of Notre Dame P, 1989.

Krueger, Frank. Kevin McCabe, Jorge Moll, Nikolaus Kriegeskorte, Roland Zahn, Maren Strenziok, Armin Heinecke, and Jordan Grafman. "Neural Correlates of Conditional and Unconditional trust in Two-Person reciprocal Exchange." *PNAS* (Proceedings of the National Academy of Sciences of the United States of America) 104.50 (2007): 20084–20089.

Lakoff, George and Mark Johnson. *Metaphors We Live By.* Chicago: U of Chicago P, 1980.

Lamm, Claus., Daniel Batson, and Jean Decety. "The Neural Substrate of Human Empathy: Effects of Perspective-taking and Cognitive Appraisal." *Journal of Cognitive Neuroscience* 19.1 (2007): 42–58.

Landau, Aaron. "No settled senses of the world can match the pleasure of that madness: The Politics of Unreason in *The Winter's Tale.*" *Cahiers Elizabethains* 64 (2003): 29–42.

Ledoux, Joseph. *The Emotional Brain: The Mysterious Underpinnings of Emotional Life.* London: Weidenfeld and Nicolson, 1998.

Lhermitte, F. M., B. Pillion, and M. Serdrau. "Human Autonomy and the Frontal Lobes. Part I: Imitation and Utilization Behavior: a Neuropsychological Study of 75 Patients." *Annals of Neurology* 19.4 (1986): 326–334.

Leverage, Paula. Howard Mancing, Richard Schweikert, and Jennifer Marston William. *Theory of Mind and Literature.* West Lafayette: Purdue UP, 2011.

Levine, Richard A. ed. *Backgrounds to Victorian Literature.* San Francisco: Chandler Publishing, 1967.

Levy, Jonathan. "A Note on Empathy." *New Ideas in Psychology* 15.2 (1997): 179–184.

Lim, Walter S. H. "Knowledge and Belief in *The Winter's Tale.*" *Studies in English Literature 1500–1900.* 41.2 (2001): 317–334.

Livingston, M. and D. Hubel. "Segregation of Form, Color, Movement, and Depth: Anatomy, Physiology, and Perception." *Science* 240.4853 (1988): 740–749.

Locke, John. *Two Treatises of Government* and *A Letter Concerning Toleration. Rethinking the Western Tradition: John Locke.* ed. Ian Shapiro. New Haven: Yale UP, 2003.

Lyotard, Jean-Francois. "Answering the Question: What is Postmodernism?" *Critique* 419 (1982). Rpt. *Modernism / Postmodernism.* Ed and int. Peter Brooker. London: Longman, 1992. 139–150.

Mackenzie, Ian. "Tom Stoppard: The Monological Imagination" *Modern Drama* 32 (1989): 574–586.

Malekin, Peter and Ralph Yarrow. *Consciousness' Literature and Theatre: Theory and Beyond.* London: Macmillan P, 1997.

Margolis, Joseph. "The Nature and Strategies of Relativism." *Mind*, New Series 92.368 (1983): 548–567.

Matheson, Carl and Evan Kirchoff. "Chaos and Literature." *Philosophy and Literature* 21.1 (1997): 28–45.

Maves, C. E. "A Playwright on the Side of Rationality." *Palo Alto Times*, March, 25, 1977. Rpt. Delaney, Paul ed. *Tom Stoppard In Conversation*. Ann Arbor: U of Michigan P, 1994. 100–102.

McConachie, Bruce. *Engaging Audiences: A Cognitive Approach to Spectating in the Theatre*. New York: Palgrave Macmillan, 2008.

Meyer, Kinereth. "It Is Written': Tom Stoppard and The Drama of The Intertext". *Comparative Drama* 23.2 (1989): 105–122.

Miller, Owen. "Intertextual Identity." *The Identity of the Literary Text*. ed. Mario J. Valdes and Owen Miller. Toronto: U of Toronto P, 1985. 19–40.

Miller, Tyrus. "Avant-Garde and Theory: A Misunderstood Relation." *Poetics Today* 20.4 (1999): 549–579.

Miller, William Ian. *The Anatomy of Disgust*. London: Harvard UP, 1997.

Milward, Peter. "A Theology of Grace in *The Winter's Tale*." *English Literature and Language* 2. 1964. 27–50. Rpt. in *The Medieval Dimension in Shakespeare's Plays. Studies in Renaissance Literature* Vol. 7. New York: Edwin Mellen, 1990. 102–124.

Moll, Jorge, Ricardo de Oliveira-Souza, Fernanda Tovar Moll, Fátima Azevedo Ignácio, Ivanei E. Bramati, Egas M. Caparelli-Dáquer, and Paul J. Eslinger."The Moral Affiliations of Disgust: A Functional MRI Study." *Cognitive Behavioral Neurology* 18.1 (2005): 68–78.

Monlar-Szakacs, Istvan, Jonas Kaplan, Patricia M. Greenfield, and Marco Iacobaoni. "Observing Complex Action Sequences: The role of the fronto-parietal mirror neuron system." *NeuroImage* 33 (2006): 923–935.

Naismith, Bill. Int. and notes to *Our County's Good* (1988). London: Methuen, 1995.

Niedenthal, Paula M., Lawrence W. Barsalou, Francois Ric, and Sylvia Krauth- Gruber, "Embodiment in the Acquisition and Use of Emotion Knowledge." *Emotion and Consciousness*. Ed. Lisa Feldman Barret, Paula M. Niedenthal and Pioter Winkielman. New York: Guilford Press, 2005.

Nietzsche, Friedrich. *The Birth of Tragedy* (1872). Rpt. in full in *The Birth of Tragedy and Other Writings*. Eds. Raymond Geuss and Ronald Speirs. Trans. Ronald Speirs. Cambridge: Cambridge UP, 1999.

———. *On the Genealogy of Morals* (1887). *Basic Writings of F. Nietzsche*. Trans. and ed. Walter Kaufman. Random House, 1966.

———. *Twilight of the Idols* (1889). Rpt in full in *The Portable Nietzsche*. ed. and trans. Walter Kaufmann (1954). New York: Viking Penguin, 1982. pp. 463–563.

———. *Thus Spoke Zarathustra* (1891). Rpt in full in *The Portable Nietzsche*. ed. and trans. Walter Kaufmann (1954). New York: Viking Penguin, 1982. pp. 103–343.

Nietzsche, Friedrich. *The Will To Power* (1901). *Great Books and Classics*: Athenaeum Library of Philosophy. http://www.grtbooks.com/nietzsche .asp?idx=3&yr=1895#power

Norris, Christopher. *The Truth About Postmodernism*. Oxford: Blackwell, 1993.

Olatunji, Bunami O., David F. Tolin, Craig N. Sawchuk, Nathan L. Williams, Jonathan S. Abramowitz, Jeffrey M. Lohr, and Lisa S. Elwood. "The Disgust Scale: Item Analysis, Factor Structure, and Suggestions for Refinement." *Psychological Assessment* 19.3 (2007): 281–297.

Orgel, Stephen. "The Poetics of Incomprehensibility." *Shakespeare Quarterly* 42.4 (1991): 431–437.

Orlich, Ileana Alexandra. "Tom Stoppard's *Travesties* and the Politics of Earnestness." *East European Quarterly* 38.3 (2004): 371–383.

Palmer, Daryl W. "Jacobean Moscovites: Winter, Tyranny, and Knowledge in *The Winter's Tale*." *Shakespeare Quarterly* 46.3 (1995): 323–339.

Paslick, Robert H. Trans. and Int. *Literature And Philosophy in Dialogue: Essays in German Literary Theory by Hans-Georg Gadamar*. Albany: State U of New York P, 1994.

Pearce, Howard D. "Stage as Mirror: Tom Stoppard's Travesties." *MLN* 94.5 (1979): 1139–1158.

Perl, Jeffrey M. *Skepticism and Modern Enmity*. Baltimore and London: Johns Hopkins UP, 1989.

Phillip, Arthur. *The Voyage of Governor Phillip to Botany Bay*. London: John Stockwell of Piccadilly, 1789.

Phillips, Mary L., Leanne M. Williams, Maike Heining, Cathrine M. Herba, Tamara Russel, Christopher Andrew, Ed T. Bullmore, Michael J. Brammer, Steven C. R. Williams, Michael Morgan, Andrew W. Young, and Jeffrey A. Gray. "Differential Neural responses to Overt and Covert Presentations of Facial Expressions of Fear and Disgust." *NeuroImage* 21 (2004): 1484–1496.

Poland, Warren S. "The Limits of Empathy." Clinician's Corner: *American Imago* 64.1 (2007): 87–93.

Premack, David and Ann James Premack. "Origins of Human Social Competence." *The Cognitive Neurosciences*. Ed. Michael S. Gazzaniga. Cambridge: MIT P., 1995.

Reddy, William M. "Sentimentalism and Its Erasure: The Role of Emotions in the Era of the French Revolution." *The Journal of Modern History* 72 (2000): 109–152.

Reinhard Lupton, Julia. *Afterlives of the Saints: Hagiography, Typology, and Renaissance Literature*. Stanford: Stanford UP, 1996.

Richardson, Alan. "Studies in Literature and Cognition: A Field Map." *The Work of Fiction: Cognition, Culture, and Complexity*. Eds. Alan Richardson and Ellen Spolsky. Aldershot: Ashgate, 2004. 1–29.

Richardson Brian. "Voice and Narration in Postmodern Drama." *New Literary History* 32.3 (2001): 681–694.

Rizzolatti Giacomo. "The mirror neuron system and its function in humans." *Anat Embryo*. 210.5–6 (2005): 419–21.

Rizzolatti, Giacomo and Michael A. Arbib. "Language Within Our Grasp." *Trends in Neuroscience* 21 (1998): 188–194.

Rizzolatti Giacomo and Laila Craighero. "The Mirror Neuron System." *Annu. Rev. Neurosci.* 27 (2004): 169–92.

Rizzolatti, Giacommo and Corrado Sinigaglia. *Mirrors in the Brain: How Our Minds Share Action and Emotion* [Italian 2006]. Trans. Frances Anderson. Oxford UP, 2008.

Robles-Pérez, Salvador, Y. Hassouni, and Pedro .F. Gonzáles-Diaz. "Coherent States in the Quantum Multiverse." *Physics Letters B* 683 (2010): 1–6.

Rokotnitz, Naomi. "Constructing Cognitive Scaffolding through Embodied Receptiveness: Toni Morrison's *The Bluest Eye*." *Style* 41.4 (2008): 385–408.

———. "'Too far gone in disgust': Mirror Neurons and the Manipulation of Embodied Responses in *The Libertine*." *Configurations* 16.3 (2010) 400–426.

Ronk, Martha, "Recasting Jealousy: A Reading of *The Winter's Tale*.," *Literature and Psychology.* 36.1–2 (1990): 50–77.

Rorty, Richard. "Deconstruction and Circumvention." *Critical Inquiry* 11.1 (1984): 1–23.

———. "Pragmatism, Relativism and Irrationalism." *Consequences of Pragmatism (Essays 197–-1980).* U of Minnesota P, 1982. 166–8.

Ross, Charlotte. *Primo Levi's Narratives of Embodiment: Containing the Human.* London: Routledge, 2011.

Rousseau, Jean-Jacques. *The Social Contract and Discourses.* Trans. G. D. H. Cole 1913. Revised and augmented by Brumfitt and Hall. London: J. M. Dent and Sons, 1973.

Sammels, Neil. "Earning Liberties: *Travesties* and *The Importance of Being Earnest*" *Modern Drama* 29.3 (1986): 376–387.

Sartre, Jean-Paul. *Being and Nothingness: An Essay on Phenomenologicasl Ontology* (1943). Trans. Hazel E. Barnes. NY: Washington Square Press, 1966.

Schank, Roger. *Tell Me a Story.* New York: Charles Scribner's Sons, 1990.

Schechner, Richard. *Performance Theory.* New York and London: Routledge, 1988.

———. "Invasions Friendly and Unfriendly: The Dramaturgy of Direct Theatre." *Critical Theory and Performance.* ed. Janelle G. Reinelt and Joseph R. Roach. Ann Arbor: U of Michigan P, 1992.

Schechner, Richard. "Performance As a 'Formation of Power and Knowledge.'" *The Drama Review* 44.4 (2002): 5–7.

———. "Rasaesthetics." *The Drama Review* 45.3 (2001): 27–50.

Schiller, Friedrich. "Ode to Joy" (1785). http://raptusassociation.org /ode1785.html

Scholes, Robert. *Protocols of Reading.* New Haven: Yale UP, 1989.

Searle, John. "The Mystery of Consciousness Continues." *The NY Review of Books* 58.10 June 2-22, 2011, pp. 50–52.

Servan-Schreiber, David. *Healing Without Freud or Prozac.* London: Rodale, 2004. First published in French, Paris: Lafont, 2003.

Shakespeare, William. *The Winter's Tale*. (1610–11). ed. Frank Kermode. The Signet Classic Shakespeare. Gen. Ed. Sylvan Barnet. Harmondsworth: Penguin, 1963.

Shelley, Percy Bysshe. *A Defense of Poetry* (1840). *Shelley's Poetry and Prose: A Norton Critical Edition*. Eds. Donald H. Reiman ansd Neil Fraistat. NY: Norton, 2002.

Showalter, Elaine. "Critical Cross-Dressing" *Raritan* 3.2 (1983): 130–149.

Silverman, Michael E., and Arien Mack. "Change Blindness and Priming: When it Does and Does Not Occur." *Consciousness and Cognition* 15 (2006): 409–422.

Singer, Tanya, Ben Seymour, John O'Doherty, Holger Kaube, Raymond J. Dolan, and Chris D. Firth. "Empathy for pain involves the affective but not the sensory components of pain." *Science* 303 (2004): 1157–1162.

Singer, Tanya and Claus Lamm. "The Social Neuroscience of Empathy." *The Year in Cognitive Neuroscience 2009: Annals of the New York Academy of Science* 1156 (2009): 81–96.

Smith, Adam. *The Theory of Moral Sentiments* (1759). Vol. I of *The Glasgow Edition of the Works and Correspondence of Adam Smith*. Eds. Raphael, David Daiches and Alec Lawrence Macfie. Indianapolis: Liberty Fund, 1982. The online edition is published by Liberty Fund under license from Oxford University Press: at http://oll.libertyfund.org/index.php?option=com_staticxt&staticfile=show.php%3Ftitle=192&layout=html#chapter_200027

———. *The Wealth of Nations* (1776). Harmonsworth: Penguin Books, 1982.

Solomon, Maynard. *Late Beethoven: Music, Thought, Imagination*. Berkeley, Los Angeles: U of California P, 2003.

Sorensen, Roy A. "Self-Strengthening Empathy." *Philosophy and Phenomenological Research* 43.2 (1998): 75–98.

Spolsky, Ellen. *Gaps in Nature: Literary Interpretation and the Modular Mind*. Albany NY: State U of New York P, 1993.

———. "Darwin and Derrida: Cognitive Literary Theory as a Species of Post-Structuralism." *Poetics Today* 23.1 (2001b): 43–62.

———. "Why and How to Take the Fruit and Leave the Chaff." *SubStance* 30.1–2 (2001c): 177–198.

———. *Satisfying Skepticism: Embodied Knowledge in the Early Modern Period*. Aldershot: Ashgate, 2001a.

States, Bert O. "The Phenomenological Attitude." *Critical Theory and Performance*. ed. Janelle G. Reinelt and Joseph R. Roach. Ann Arbor: U of Michigan P, 1992.

———. "Dreams: The Royal Road to Metaphor." *SubStance* 30.1–2 (2001): 104–118.

Stoppard, Tom. *Travesties*. 1975. New York: Grove, 1976.

Sullivan, Esther Beth. "Hailing Ideology, Acting in the Horizon, and Reading Between Plays by Timberlake Wertenbaker." *Theater Journal* 43.2 (1993): 139–154.

Tegmark, Max. "Parallel Universes." *Science and Ultimate Reality: From Quantum to Cosmos*, honoring John Wheeler's 90th birthday. Eds. J. D. Barrow, P. C. W. Davies, and C. L. Harper. Cambridge: Cambridge UP, 2003.

Talmon, Jacob Leib. *Romanticism and Revolution: Europe 1815–1848*. Harcourt, Brace & World, INC, 1967.

Tench, Watkin. *Sydney's First Four Years* (Including *A Narrative of the Expedition To Botany Bay* (1788) and *A Complete Account of the Settlement at Port Jackson* (1793). Int. L. F. Fitzharding. Sydney: Angus and Robertson, 1961.

Thatcher, David, "Begging to Differ: Modes of Discrepancy in Shakespeare," *Studies in Shakespeare 8*. Gen. ed. R. F. Willson, Jr. New York: Peter Lang, 1999.

Thomas Crane, Mary. "What Was Performance?" *Criticism* 43.2 (2001): 169–187.

Traub, Valerie, "Jewels, Statues, and Corpses: Containment of Female Erotic Power (*Hamlet, Othello, The Winter's Tale*)." *Desire and Anxiety: Circulation of Sexuality In Shakespearean Drama*. New York: Routledge, 1992, 25–50.

Turner, Stephen. "Imitation or the Internalization of Norms: is Twentieth Century Social Theory Based on the Wrong Choice?" *Empathy and Agency*. eds. and int. Hans Herbert Kögler and Karsten R. Steuber. Boulder: Westview, 2000. 103–118.

Umilta, Maria Alessandra, Evelyne Kohler, Vittorio Gallese, Leonardo Fogassi, Luciano Fadiga, Chrisdtian Keysers, and Giaccomo Rizolatti. "I Know What You Are Doing—A Neuropsychological Study." *Neuron* 31.1 (2001): 155–65.

Vanden Heuvel, Michael. "'Is Postmodernism?': Stoppard Among/Against the Postmoderns." *The Cambridge Companion to Tom Stoppard*. Ed. Kathrine E. Kelly. Cambridge: Cambridge UP, 2001.

Varela, Francisco J., Evan Thompson, and Eleanor Rosch, *The Embodied Mind: Cognitive Science and Human Experience*. Cambridge, MA: MIT Press, 1991.

Walker, Charles. *The Encyclopedia of Secret Knowledge*. London: Random House, 1995.

Walker, Julia A. "Why Performance? Why Now? Textuality and the Rearticulation of Human Presence." *The Yale Journal of Criticism* 16.1 (2003): 149–175.

Weeks, Stephen. "The Question of Liz: Staging the Prisoner in *Our Country's Good*." *Modern Drama* 43.2 (2000): 147–157.

Wertenbaker, Timberlake. *Our County's Good* (1988). Int. and notes Bill Naismith. London: Methuen, 1995.

———. Preface to the program for the production at The Young Vic Theatre, October 22, 1998, directed by Max Stafford-Clark.

Wetzsteon, Ross. "Tom Stoppard Eats Steak Tartare with Chocolate Sauce" (1975). Rpt. *Tom Stoppard In Conversation*. ed. Paul Delaney. Ann Arbor: U of Michigan P, 1994. 80–84.

Wilde, Oscar. *The Picture of Dorian Gray* (1890). *The Complete Stories, Plays and Poems of Oscar Wilde*. London: Tiger Books International, 1990. 11–161.

———. *The Critic As Artist* (1891). *The Norton Anthology of English Literature II*. 8th ed. Eds. Stephen Greenblatt and M.H. Abrams. New York: W.W. Norton & Co., 2006.

———. *The Importance of Being Earnest*. *The Complete Stories, Plays and Poems of Oscar Wilde*. London: Tiger Books International, 1990. 315–363.

Wilson, Ann. "*Our Country's Good*: Theatre, Colony and Nation in Wertenbaker's Adaptation of *The Playmaker*." *Modern Drama*. 34.1 (1991) 23–32.

Worthen, W. B. "Drama, Performativity and Performance." *PMLA* 113.5 (1998): 1093–1107.

Young, Kay and Jeffrey L. Saver. "The Neurology of Narrative." *SubStance* 30.1–2 (2001): 72–84.

Zak, Michail. "Complexity for Survival of livings." *Chaos, Solitions and Fractals* 32 (2007): 1154–1167.

Zamir, Tzachi. *Double Vision*. Princeton: Princeton UP, 2007.

Zinman, Toby. "*Travesties, Night and Day, The Real Thing*." *The Cambridge Companion to Tom Stoppard*. Ed. Kathrine E. Kelly. Cambridge: Cambridge UP, 2001.

Zuckow-Goldring, Patricia and Michael Arbib. "Affordances, Effectivities, and Assisted Imitation: Caregivers and the Directing of Attention." *Neurocomputing* 70 (2007): 2181–2193.

Zunshine, Lisa. "Theory of Mind and Experimental Representations of Fictional Consciousness." *Narrative* 11.3 (2003): 270–291.

Index

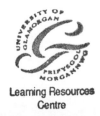